Revelations
on
Healing

Revelations
on
Healing

·······

*What One Doctor
Discovered Channeling
Messages for His Patients*

PETER WISCH, M.D.

**TURNING
STONE
PRESS**

Cover design by Peter Wisch
Cover art by Peter Wisch
Interior Design by Howie Severson

Turning Stone Press
8301 Broadway Street, Suite 219
San Antonio, TX 78209
www.turningstonepress.com

Library of Congress Control Number
is available upon request.

ISBN 978-1-61852-130-9

Printed in the United States of America

This book is dedicated to
Kerianne Desiderio.
My journey of healing
could not have been possible without her.
She is a fountain of light and love,
bound forever to my soul and to my heart
and throughout the pages of this book.

Contents

Disclaimer

A significant point to keep in mind as you read this book is that in no way do I deny or renounce any of the traditional or unconventional forms of treatment. I support any form of healing whose intent is to benefit without causing harm. I offer the ideologies of healing presented in this book to be utilized as adjunctive therapies, albeit powerful and potent ones in the complex and diverse menu of available therapeutic options.

Unless otherwise noted, the case studies in this book refer to authentic individuals. Many are patients, acquaintances, or friends. The stories are honest accounts of portions of their lives, although their names and some of the details have been changed to protect their identities. Some accounts are derived from notable media items and public figures.

Introduction

A New View and Way of Healing

As a healer from a conventional medical background, I have always felt that there were fundamental gaps in the prevailing comprehensive understanding of disease and healing. I found it insufficient that patients were routinely diagnosed and treated without exploring or uncovering the deeper reasons for their conditions that could potentially offer more insight and benefit to not only alleviate but also cure and prevent illness. Labeling conditions with exotic designations, prescribing complex medications, and excising demonstrative bodily growths did not seem adequate. I felt that there must be more to healing than just that.

Having practiced dermatology for close to twenty-nine years, I was often asked numerous seemingly basic and sincere medical questions by patients desperate for vital knowledge for which my responses felt ineffectual and unsatisfactory. For instance, when a patient with a drug rash resulting from a hypersensitivity reaction to penicillin asked me why their body had manifested such an allergy, I could certainly explain that reaction on a chemical, immunological, physiological, and pharmacological level. However, did any of that information truly serve the patient? That void of meaningful and edifying therapeutic knowledge plagued my mind for years. I felt impotent as a healer dispensing scientific jargon to a patient the same way a lawyer uses incomprehensible and perplexing legal terminology with a client. My technical language was covering up a more profound wisdom I had not yet discovered. If I were ever going to be the healer I strived to be, I had to persevere in my quest to learn the mysteries of healing that were eluding me. I, like many of my patients, longed to know meaningful explanations and fundamental truths.

I did eventually and wondrously come upon some profound answers to many of those pivotal mystifying quandaries regarding healing, and the way that came about was quite intriguing and remarkable. I was introduced to a discipline called channeling, whereby in altering my own state of consciousness I have been able to connect with an expanded one that instills me with a most illuminating and wise source of information. Through this practice, my fund of knowledge regarding healing has grown in ways that I relished yet could not have imagined. Much of what I became aware of were simple and yet basic age-old truths that did not negate but instead harmonized with and complemented many modern technological advancements. I shared many of these insights, albeit in a much more focused and personal nature, with patients, friends, and family members when I felt it was appropriate and could be beneficial to their particular troubles. I was often pleasantly surprised by the results. As I pressed on with my new awareness, my experiences, abilities, and knowledge base grew further. I was becoming more like the healer I wanted to be, and

I felt that I was making a more meaningful difference in my patients' lives.

Since one of the most basic needs common to everyone is the desire to heal and because of all the valuable knowledge concerning health and healing that had come upon me, I decided to write this book in order to share my newfound enlightenment with a larger audience. The subject matter emanates from my heart; healing has always been a deep and sacred passion of mine professionally as well as personally. The principles I cover can apply to anyone, and I truly believe that they are paramount to healing.

This book, which offers a more comprehensive meaning of the nature of healing, presents a powerful, essential, and enlightening message: all four dimensions of your being—the body, the mind, the emotions, and the spirit—are inexorably linked to total wellness. How each dimension functions, how it supports healing, and how best to approach it are explored. Additionally, it demonstrates how you can uncover answers, insights, and truths to assist you in taking control and generating your own health and vitality through the information, case histories, and exercises presented. It explains how the forces of change influence healing and how you can affect those forces in ways that can most benefit you. And ultimately, it elucidates how you can contribute in a comprehensible, straightforward, and intrinsic way to global healing.

To grasp more clearly how I arrived on this distinctive course, it would be helpful to know about some serendipitous events that occurred in my life around the early to mid-1990s that guided me in this direction. During that time, in the course of treating patients several evocative and affirming events awakened my psyche, foreshadowing my own transformative journey.

First, my experiences treating a couple made me keenly aware of an issue I needed to find a better way to manage: not only did some patients conceal pertinent information from their doctors, but also were dishonest with themselves. I treated a husband and wife separately and unbeknownst to the other, and I did not divulge any information revealed to me from one to the other. During the wife's examination, she railed about the problems in her marriage and disclosed that she had recently served her husband with divorce papers. Shortly thereafter the husband came to see me for an uncomfortable rash that I felt was unequivocally due to excess tension. When I questioned him about that possibility, he answered, "I have no stress in my life." You do not have to be a mind reader to know that anyone making that kind of blanket statement is either intentionally hiding something or is in utter denial. After these events I wondered if there could be a way to be privy to the deepest, most hidden, and most truthful contents of someone's mind in order to help them heal more completely and effectively!

It was before two remarkable incidents with patients and during a dark, turbulent, and dispirited period in my personal life when a light reached out to me and provided me with a new and illuminating perspective on healing. I was finding little solace from the more conventional sources of guidance when a friend recommended I consult a counselor who specialized in channeling. With her tools, gifts, and wisdom, this healer offered me clarity, insight, hope, and guidance and was able to delve much more accurately and expeditiously into the true origins of my problems than anyone I had previously consulted.

This novel and yet unorthodox practice helped me find my way out of the darkness. I was grateful for and captivated by this unusual and extraordinary form of healing. I not only desired to know more about it but needed to be a part of it. I was determined to assimilate all the knowledge and proficiency I could. Fortuitously, this gifted counselor was also teaching her craft and agreed to take me on as a pupil. That training period lasted two and a half years.

There is an old adage, "When the student is ready, the teacher appears," but in my case there were several teachers. Concurrently and shortly after my first mentor, I connected with and studied under three other learned ones in that genre. Each had a unique style of tutelage as well as philosophy regarding the subject matter. I felt blessed to be exposed to all this. The last teacher was indeed a special gift from the Universe. Not only was she a wise mentor and role model to me, but she also became a great friend and colleague. I was fortunate to have had the opportunity to work with her conducting several group healing workshops and retreats. And when she finally retired from her channeling practice, I felt privileged and honored that she decided to refer her clients to me.

After I had established myself in this new passion, two other mind-altering incidents with patients occurred that reaffirmed my dedication to my newfound progressive course. One happened one summer weekend morning while I was covering for another physician on holiday. I received a call from his service that one of his patients was experiencing a severe case of hives. I rang up the patient. She informed me that the rash had persisted for three days despite her taking a popular over-the-counter antihistamine. I took an extensive medical history from her over the phone, which included a complete review of all her systems. The patient answered no to everything that could possibly be implicated as a cause of her symptoms.

Before setting up an appointment to see her that morning, I asked her to hold the line for one moment while I went to check something. I closed my eyes, took several deep breaths, and in a quasi-meditative state of consciousness channeled my Higher Wisdom, asking for guidance regarding what else I needed to know that would serve my highest good to help heal this woman. Shortly thereafter a vision appeared in my mind of a torrential downpour, but the odd thing was that the rain was a golden yellow color. I then asked my Higher Wisdom if this woman was having a urinary tract infection. I heard a resounding, "Affirmative!" I wondered if that was the source of her hives. Again, the response was clearly, "Affirmative!"

When I got back on the phone, I asked the woman a second time about any urinary symptoms she might be experiencing. She timidly responded that about two weeks before she had had a full-fledged urinary tract infection and had called her gynecologist, who prescribed a course of antibiotics. She did not bother to finish taking all the capsules because her symptoms had dissipated after a few days. During the past week, she had again started to experience some mild intermittent urinary symptoms, but they did not seem severe enough for her to consider seeking any treatment. I asked why she had not told me about those symptoms when I had specifically questioned her about them earlier, and she replied that she was embarrassed to tell me since she did not know me well and she did not see how a problem with her bladder could possibly be related to her rash. I told her that

I thought it was absolutely relevant. One of the major causes of hives is infection. I instructed her to call her internist or gynecologist and tell them about her urinary symptoms. Once that problem is resolved, I told her, her skin condition should dissipate.

That incident revealed to me that channeling could help me uncover specific physical causes for illness. However, over the course of my many other experiences utilizing channeling to help heal patients, I discovered there were more profound reasons for medical illnesses than just physical causes—factors over which patients have a great deal more control than they are aware.

The next incident demonstrated this insight to me. I saw a young woman in her mid-thirties with a severe case of dyshidrosis, a rare type of eczema primarily limited to the palms and soles and often induced by acute emotional stress. She presented with both ruptured oozing and intact blisters, swelling, redness, intractable itching, considerable discomfort, and a secondary bacterial infection on her palms and fingers. This woman had been experiencing episodes of this nature approximately every three to four months for about a year. She responded favorably to treatment with antibiotics, corticosteroids, and lukewarm astringent compresses.

On a follow-up visit, she asked me why she kept experiencing this condition. I explained that quite often severe anxiety is responsible for physical maladies such as the one affecting her. I asked her what she thought the cause could possibly be. She stared at me cluelessly. Instead of giving her the technical medical explanation, which I did not feel would be helpful nor would she comprehend, I simply channeled what she needed to know about the breakout on her hands.

The information I received shocked her. I told her that I knew how desperately she wanted to get married, but the man she has been dating for the past several years was not capable of making a commitment of that sort. It was highly unlikely she was ever going to get the engagement ring that she so yearned for from him. I told her that if she really wanted to get married to someone who truly loved her enough to commit to her, she should leave this man and set higher standards for herself. Her self-esteem was low; she needed to do some work in that area, possibly in therapy. One of the reasons she had attracted this unappreciative man into her life was so that she would be compelled to confront her self-worth issues. On a rational level, she knew deep inside that this man was not going to marry her, but she still hoped and dreamed otherwise. Her hands were sending her a clear and powerful message: "No engagement ring is ever going to fit comfortably on that swollen, red, and blistering conjugal finger!"

She looked at me as if I had come from outer space and asked, "How do you know all this about me? Have you been speaking to my mother?"

All my new knowledge was propelling me toward integrating this exciting revelatory and yet unconventional adjunct to healing with the best of what already existed. I was at a crossroads where I needed to discover, explore, and assimilate as much of this newfound discipline of channeling as possible in order to move forward. What I have learned through my experiences I now share with you in this book so that you too may also reap its benefit and heal. The healing messages are universal truths which I have channeled from an enlightened source to address everyone (including me)—from now on collectively referred to throughout the book as "you."

Lastly, I have no doubt that some of my words will elicit controversy and incredulity. I believe that a dose of skepticism as well as broad-mindedness regarding any innovative and recondite construct is healthy and that it can stimulate people to think and ideas to grow. I wholeheartedly support anything that leads to well-being, no matter where it comes from as long as it is of virtuous and beneficent intent and does no harm. After all, if you have your health, you possess your most invaluable asset. And if in writing this book, I guide anyone to heal, I shall have accomplished what I set out to do.

❧ 1 ❧

The Nature of Healing

Understanding Healing

During your life span, you have a multitude of opportunities for healing, although you may not often view them that way. When you wander too far off course from your natural proclivities, your innate yearnings in life, or the rightful purpose that drew you to this existence, you may notice signs of personal instability and disruption; your physical body, your emotions, or your rational mind can become unhealthy, unstable, or ill at ease. Some of you choose to ignore the signs and symptoms of affliction, hoping that they will miraculously dissipate. It is like a car engine that is starting to fail. If you ignore the conking sound, it will persist until the din eventually escalates and the motor stalls on the freeway.

Through indicators of disease, healing forces beckon you to make changes and find solutions. These alterations are what help to align all your composite life-sustaining systems with your willfully chosen fundamental life purpose. I have heard more than once from recovered cancer patients that being faced with the harrowing diagnosis of cancer actually became a turning point in their lives that eventually evolved into a blessing in disguise. At first I was puzzled by that reasoning, but now I understand what those individuals meant. The impact of receiving the diagnosis of cancer forced them to step back, reevaluate their lives, and make the necessary and often huge changes to return to their true path. For an illness like cancer, you might have to make modifications that are sometimes massive, such as switching careers or leaving a marriage or forgiving a parent for childhood abuse. Healing in such cases usually involves altering a previously firmly held mental paradigm or releasing pernicious emotions or carrying out a constructive life-transforming act coupled with conventional treatments like surgery, chemotherapy, or radiotherapy in addition to adopting beneficial lifestyle changes such as a healthy diet and exercise program. Not all healing requires such extreme measures, but in every case you are called to make an adjustment or realignment of some sort in order to get back on track.

It should be rather apparent to you now that the definition of *healing* is often much more profound and encompassing than procuring a remedy for a symptom like consuming an aspirin to soothe a headache. Not only does healing deal with optimal ways to relieve discomfort and suffering, but it also comprises the wondrous journey of growing and evolving into the whole perfect individual you innately are—finding yourself; for whom you are striving to become, in actuality is who you already by nature are. Peeling away the masks and protective and obscuring layers that conceal your essence, beauty, and truth is a fundamental part of what constitutes your journey of healing in this lifetime.

Healing is complex and permeates many dimensions—physical, mental, emotional, and spiritual—all intricately and carefully intertwined. Each dimension has a significant impact in defining your uniqueness and maintaining or restoring your total health. Because treating one area has an effect on another, it is best to look at the whole entity and not focus solely on individual parts or systems. It is like when a leak appears in your wall: instead of just repairing the plaster and paint, it is more prudent to investigate the problem more thoroughly. Perhaps the trouble stems from a leaking pipe inside the wall or possibly beyond that point such as escalating pressure in the water tank. Do not just deal with superficial annoyances, but search for, find, and remedy the trouble at its core. The same holds true with human beings: besides just dealing with the symptom, go to the source of the matter no matter how deep or concealed it might seem to be. That headache mentioned earlier might have had at its origin a more complex physical problem such as high blood pressure and perhaps even something deeper such as an emotional stressor of a financial or romantic nature. The aspirin might have helped temporarily, but if the headache recurs, probing deeper may be the best way to restore balance and feel better again—to find and work on the ultimate responsible source behind the symptom.

Healing on Different Levels

One of the biggest misconceptions is that healing exclusively or predominantly applies to the physical body. That is because in your world, the major emphasis on healing is concerned with bodily health. After all, you live in a physical dimension; for the most part, you cannot see, hear, smell, taste, or touch your emotions, thoughts, or soul. You generally go to a doctor for a physical examination. Whether the reason is an annual checkup or because you are complaining of some dysfunction or ache, either the health care provider or the patient traditionally focuses on the corporeal aspects. The doctor customarily takes a thorough history regarding the various systems of the body and then proceeds to examine the body. He or she may then order and subsequently analyze results from some physical tests such as x-rays, biopsies, and blood and urine samples before rendering an assessment and recommending a plan.

Yet you are not just a physical body but are composed of three other essential elements. You have access to a whole range of mental, emotional, and spiritual resources for healing. To console and counsel your spiritual side, there is no dearth of clergy or advisors affiliated with churches, temples, mosques, ashrams, spiritual societies, or any number of faith-based traditions. There is also a whole segment of the health care community comprising psychiatrists, psychologists, social workers, etc., to specifically deal with mental and emotional issues.

The mind, the emotions, and the soul are abstract and more complex and challenging for you to sense, but you must strive to heal on all four constituents of your being. Those four linked dimensions are like a bunch of helium balloons, each with its own attached string tied to a common knot. Each balloon is continuously attempting to raise itself and help lift the other three toward a zenith—its optimum state of health. If just one of those constituents or balloons is weighed down by malady or impairment, the entire set will be hindered from rising to reach peak levels. Until you learn to heal yourselves on all four planes of physical, cognitive, emotional, and spiritual well-being, you will never attain your highest point of healthy development. Since you primarily regard yourselves as physical beings inhabiting a physical reality, it is understandable that you tend to equate health with physical vitality. But the physical body is just one vehicle, albeit a prime constituent, that you have been entrusted with to help you navigate throughout your life. The mind, emotions, and soul are equally important and often neglected genuine components of your being. They are certainly more abstract and amorphous when compared to the tangible physical realm, but that does not mean they are not as essential and valuable to your health. Those aspects of your being actually persist beyond the physical body's span, so it is essential to fully engage with them in order to feel whole and make your journey in the physical dimension optimal.

While so many resources for healing are available, whether they address the physical, mental, emotional, or spiritual aspects of what plagues you, the issue for many is not knowing the true origin of a problem and essentially how and where to begin healing. Yes, you can always start by treating the symptom, but what if a headache that initially responded to aspirin recurs? There is certainly a physical aberration to analyze and treat, but beyond that, there is often a deeper underlying cause to investigate and address. The most challenging and yet illuminating task in evaluating the signs and symptoms of disease is to listen to the wisdom from which a body speaks. Understanding the bigger picture and knowing the more profound and true source of a disorder are key factors to healing in the most efficacious way.

Affliction Acting as a Guiding Force for Healing

Within each person there is a natural tendency toward healing—toward bringing the whole self back to a homeostatic state of well-being. One of the reasons why illness presents itself is to remind you to move toward a better path—the light, life purpose, or the place where the soul seeks greatest fulfillment. Granted, nobody wants to travel far from their optimal course, to be in a dark or lonely place and suffer, but is it not comforting to know corrective forces in the Universe exist that are designed to steer you back from where you have strayed and restore you to equanimity, solace, and hence, a healthier state? The Universe guides you or, in effect, sends you messages via your body, your mind, your soul, or your feelings and sometimes in the form of a malady, trouble, or discomfort when you have not heeded subtler signs to make modifications needed in your life. These messages essentially aim to steer you in a more optimal direction or align you with the proper energy frequencies to allow you to press on more smoothly. The trick is to learn to efficiently and effectively receive and understand these messages and act on them. As you learn to become more aware and attuned to all the diverse elements of your being, you will have a finer sense of what you need to do to be in a better place. Whatever part of you might be unhealthy—physical, mental, emotional, or spiritual—if you can view your situation as a guide and not some terrifying adversity, the experience may not be as frightening as you might have perceived it to be at one time. You merely need to rearrange your mindset regarding infirmity to allow yourself to think of it more as a corrective signal. The hardest part is to be calm, insightful, and receptive enough to take notice of what that illuminating communiqué camouflaged as affliction is trying to tell you.

Evan and his father, Jock, found out how powerful paying attention to such messages can be. Evan was a junior in high school when he first experienced bouts of major mood swings later diagnosed as bipolar disorder. His father took the news quite hard and was filled with shame and distress. Jock was a proud, driven, and accomplished physician, sailor, and skier, who had high hopes and set lofty standards for his firstborn son. Jock stressed that Evan do outstanding work in school so that he could matriculate at the "right" college and thereafter at the "right" medical school and so on. Jock also pushed Evan to excel competitively in both sailing and downhill skiing. Evan struggled to fulfill his father's aspirations, and he clearly felt intense pressure.

After experiencing a mental breakdown, Evan spent several months in an in-patient psychiatric facility where he was prescribed medications to help balance his moods and underwent counseling to seek answers and understand why these changes had occurred in his life. Always having led his life to please his strong-willed, successful, and demanding father, Evan was now powerless to do so as well as liberated from doing so. Fortunately, with the help of both individual and family counseling, father and son were able to take a fresh look at themselves and their relationship. Evan was a sensitive and emotional young man who had suppressed his true essence in order to become the man his father wanted him to be, while Jock was so formidable and headstrong he thought that he knew what was best for his son without really knowing who he was.

The bipolar disorder served as a catalyst to uncover the strain and suffering of both father and son and led them to look inside themselves, evaluate what transpired, and reestablish a new and healthier relationship. In effect, it was a blessing in disguise that awakened them to heal. It created, at first, a challenging setback and, ultimately a stable therapeutic environment, both of which were significant factors which helped them to value and accept themselves and each other so that they could both forge ahead with their own life purpose and fulfill the best of their potential. Evan went on to develop a website with a chat room for teenagers dealing with mental illness. His moods are now stable with some help from medication and therapy. He is studying psychology and business at college, where he is both the founder and president of a young entrepreneurs' club. His father is now very proud and supportive.

You Are the Creators of Your Own State of Being

I have always been intrigued by the adage, "we plan our lives, but accidents [inconveniences, afflictions] control them." But are they truly accidents? You do indeed have some responsibility in what happens. Your thoughts, actions, visualizations, procrastinations, or fears do in some way attract them. You are a creator, not a victim, of your reality. Make the effort to learn and grow from these difficulties.

It is possible to benefit from relapsing afflictions—and I do mean *benefit*. You possess your own built-in barometers—your body's signs and symptoms—that nudge you to look deeper for direction and answers. It would be ungracious and negligent to ignore them! If you could take the time to analyze how you may have created this ebb and flow in your state of well-being, you would uncover incredibly revealing explanations that would be invaluably illuminating. Way ahead of his time, Albert Schweitzer displayed how eloquently he understood the nature of healing when he stated, "The doctor of the future will be oneself."

As a dermatologist, I often saw patients annoyed with recurrent bouts of acne cysts or psoriasis or eczema, who would ask, "why me?" and "why now?" When pressed to answer for themselves, they predominately choose to look to external explanations, such as a change in either diet, detergent, cream, or climate—forsaking the complete picture. Generally the cause is due to a combination of factors. It is easier to assign blame to an outside source than to accept personal accountability, but it takes a more evolved individual to comprehend how you are responsible for creating your own circumstances regarding your health. The truth is that you do generate beneficial as well as unfavorable states. As you grow and mature, the mistakes you make as well as your positive outcomes have the potential to teach you how you can direct your energies in order to achieve vigor and wellness. It is ineffectual to assume guilt or play the role of victim for attracting affliction, but conversely empowering to know that you have the capability to evolve and create your own good state of health.

Once you are open to seeing your disorders as messages and have learned how to decode them, the next step is to act upon the advice you have gained. That can be a daunting task. It is one order, albeit trying, to comprehend the issues, but an even taller one to muster the pluck to address them. It takes a determined will and courage to do the work. The anticipation alone can be agonizing, traumatic, and unsettling. Healing is not an endeavor for the weak or the timid, but the rewards and benefits are worth all the angst and labor. Getting past the obstacle(s) responsible for the affliction can be one liberating and exhilarating experience.

Alice, a sixty-year-old wife, mother, and school-teacher, saw firsthand how empowering it was to take responsibility for her own healing by making incremental as well as instrumental changes in her life. Alice would visit my office every few months with severe flare-ups of dermatitis. She would often scratch her feet, legs, and thighs until she drew blood, and many times the abraded patches and plaques were also infected with microbes. Alice was despondent and desperate for relief, and I would provide her with the finest modern medical treatment available. Fortunately, her skin would always mend, but regrettably she would often be back with the same symptoms within a few months because the underlying source of her troubles had not gone away. In Alice's case, the allopathic treatment was merely a bandage concealing and suppressing the symptoms which were attempting to express the more profound cause of her problem. In order to heal the dermatitis at its origin, she had to delve deeper into her psyche and work with some heavy and sensitive issues.

Alice had grown up with an authoritative father. To gain his approval and love, she had been respectful and obedient and played the role of the "good little girl" exceptionally well. When she grew up, she married a man with a similar disposition, and she continued to play the same role that had worked well for her before. However, deep inside she was feeling frustrated. In one regard, she craved more pluck and independence, while on another level she feared that her husband would reject her and not support her growth and transformation.

Her repudiation of her own emerging sensibilities was beginning to take its toll on her health. Her body was prodding her to make changes. The message it was sending was that she literally needed to stand more confidently and firmly on her own two feet—the part of her anatomy by which and by no coincidence she was plagued. With guidance, Alice came to the realization that what was happening on the inside and what was manifesting on the outside were connected. Then she was able to be a more active participant in her own healing. Instead of taking giant leaps, she decided to take small steps. She gradually revealed to her husband how she felt, what she wanted to do, and who she wanted to be. Her dermatitis still recurred from time to time, but less often and less severely. Each time it reappeared it was pointing out to Alice when she had taken a step backward.

Healing with and without Assistance

You have amazing abilities to heal yourself, although there will be times when you may require assistance. No child grows and evolves without nurturing, protection, and guidance from parents, relatives, peers, teachers, and society. Whether support emanates from informal channels such as a lover or chance encounter with a stranger or through more formal arrangements such as a physician, member of the clergy, dietician, psychologist, etc., is inconsequential. No man is an island. You have all been placed in the world together to help each other thrive and survive, and there are a multitude of resources at your disposal.

The following scenarios demonstrate the roles your own resources can play in healing with and without outside assistance. Let's suppose a person suffers from a viral lung infection. If the body is otherwise in good health, is given good nourishment, handles stress satisfactorily, and gets proper rest and activity, it can often defend itself from the invader and restore the inflamed tissues of the lungs to their normal state of well-being. The symptoms of cough, fatigue, fever, sweats, chest discomfort, muscle aches, and mucous secretion will gradually abate, and the physical body will have healed without external aid. If on the other hand, the physical body was already weakened by such underlying factors like chronic obstructive pulmonary disease or one or more other conditions or medications that weaken its abilities to defend itself adequately, it might not be able to overpower the pernicious virus on its own and might require outside resources. With allies such as antiviral and other medicines, ventilators and other respiratory equipment, pulmonary therapists, nurses, physicians, and the loving support of family and friends, the physical body must work in conjunction with such assistance to try to rid the body of the hostile intruder and restore itself to its natural healthy state. Every case is different and a successful outcome is never guaranteed, but when necessary, outside assistance can certainly better the odds of healing.

Will to Live

A person must be either able and willing to do the work of healing alone or amenable and available to be assisted. If the desire to get better does not exist or cannot be encouraged or attained, there is either no or negligible hope of rehabilitation or improvement. Some people are so tormented that the thought of death might seem like a relief and a release from suffering. It is difficult but not impossible to encourage these individuals to see even a hint of light in all their darkness despite support and love from family and friends and attention by professional health care workers. Their emotions and attitudes might seem fixed as they choose to view their situation with blinders. However, if there is even a smidgen of desire for betterment, there exists a possibility for healing. It is important that all those attending to the afflicted be there for support even when a passion for living appears to be extinguished. There *can* be a change of heart or mind. It is not the end until it is the end—even though in actuality it never really is the end.

Mrs. Spolansky, a bright, refined, and gracious widow in her late seventies, lost her only son in a tragic scuba diving mishap. They were very close, and this loss affected her much more dramatically than her husband succumbing to cancer ten years earlier. She plummeted into a deep depression, and she no longer desired to carry on with her life. She terminated all social engagements and remained isolated in her large apartment to basically subsist and mourn her son's passing. She no longer paid much attention to hygiene, nutrition, and common daily rituals. Gradually she became emaciated, confined to a wheelchair, mentally unstable, and her granddaughter ultimately arranged for round-the-clock aides to attend to her basic needs. She refused any medical, psychological, or spiritual support. All she talked about was wanting to die, and within months of her son's passing, she did just that.

The will to die can take a protracted course, as in the case of Mrs. Spolansky, or a more acute time frame when a parent or spouse succumbs sometimes within minutes, hours, or days after the loss of a beloved. Reactions to such a devastation are diverse and depend on many variables like the underlying level of development and fortitude of the physical, mental, spiritual, and emotional constitution.

Despite grave or bleak prospects, more favorable out-comes can prevail if the distressed individual holds even a sliver of hope. The will to live can be quite powerful; if you alter your thoughts toward a more positive outlook, a higher vibrational level can be established that has the potential to overcome affliction. One small candle can illuminate a darkened room. The light of hope, prayer, and optimism is a mighty potent force; never underesti-mate it.

Death is not always an option. Kathy, in her early fifties, had a turbulent relationship with her father. Of all her five siblings, she was the most like him in personal-ity and temperament, yet she clashed with him until her early forties when she moved to another city to escape and deal with her own personal demons. Distance and therapy helped her to see her father in a different light. They would communicate over the phone weekly, and she would visit for about a month every summer. After so many years, they had finally developed a close, lov-ing, and compassionate bond. Approximately ten years after Kathy moved out of town, her father died from lung cancer. Of all her siblings, she took his death the hardest. Kathy's relationship with her dad had become so tight that she no longer wanted to live without him. Four weeks after he died, Kathy was diagnosed with the very same cancer her father had had in the exact same location in the same lobe of the left lung, yet at a more advanced stage. She then moved back home to be with her mother, her sisters, and friends, who encouraged and supported her to get well despite her listless, hopeless, and self-destructive attitude. Initially she begrudgingly abided by their wishes and underwent surgery and che-motherapy. Somehow with much dedication, persistence, love, and devotion, her family, friends, and health care team rallied to lift her spirits and resurrect her will to live. I am delighted to report that Kathy is now free of cancer. Her initial will to die attracted her illness, but her more potent will to live, which was subsequently uncovered and nurtured, eventually reigned triumphant.

Opening to Different Types of Healing

There exist many different sources of information, healers, and therapeutic choices when you are faced with managing a health issue. Much careful and judicious consideration must go into the decision-making process. Each treatment is unique. Some methods vary more in their degree of intensity, innovation, risk, and convention than others. Whatever option feels right to you, so be it. Metaphysically, the treatment options you feel the most trust, faith, certainty, and propitiousness toward are more likely to attract the best outcome. No one has the right to judge another person's choices concerning their own well-being, and there does not exist any one field or modality which will guarantee a 100 percent success rate. You can always benefit by being open to several options. As one of my more sagacious professors in my residency training program once told me, "If there is a disease for which the literature assigns a wide variety of treatments, odds are good that not any one of them is a sure thing!" That does not mean that there is no likelihood of a cure, but it does suggest that it might be necessary to reflect on or try out a few treatments before you discover the one that is right for you.

Since you are all composed of such diverse constitutions, no one treatment is perfect for everyone. That being the case, it makes sense to familiarize yourself with different ideologies and methodologies in order to cover a broader array of therapeutic possibilities and optimize the chance of achieving the best outcome. In other words, because not every philosophy and design of healing is a guarantee for every afflicted individual, the more comprehensive the range of therapeutic options, the greater the likelihood of matching up the most efficacious remedy with the right person.

In addition, the proper treatment may include several therapeutic choices whether consecutively, concurrently, or intermittently. For instance, working with a medical doctor, a physical therapist, and an acupuncturist, consulting a dietician, taking yoga and meditation classes, or even conferring with a trusted intuitive may be the ideal combination of healing modalities to help Carlos, who is afflicted with multiple sclerosis (MS). That regimen may not be as effective for Mabel, who also has MS. She might fare better with her medical doctor, massage therapist, herbalist, and psychologist.

The array of therapeutic choices may often seem confusing and overwhelming, especially when you may be anxious and uneducated about unfamiliar infirmities, terminologies, choices, and conventions. It is wise to do your own research as well as consult trusted sources for advice. Go to the library. Surf the internet. Speak to professionals in the appropriate fields and to people with similar conditions or get opinions from family, friends, or colleagues. But most important, *do what feels right to you*. Ultimately, it is your health, your mind, your feelings, your spirit, and your body. Never choose a healer, methodology, treatment, diet, medicine, or regimen if it does not resonate favorably at your deepest instinctual level. I once knew a widower in his eighties who was told that he needed an operation or else he might only have approximately one more year to live. He was not in favor of the surgery, but his three daughters vehemently compelled him to go forward with it. As no medical procedure is without risk, he died three days after the operation due to complications. One year can seem like an eternity compared to three days. Against his better judgment he succumbed to his daughters' demands, however well-intentioned.

Prejudgment and Healing

It is human nature to look others up and down and even sideways. You make comparisons all the time. Quite simply, you judge. It is sometimes easier and less demanding to observe and study others than to better oneself, which can take time, effort, patience, grit, determination, and some deep introspection. Whether you are following a strict diet, working out regularly at the gym, or going to a therapist weekly, these are all huge endeavors and not to be undertaken lightly. But being jealous of Jennifer because she seems to have it "all together" or berating Vincent for supposedly consuming too much food is an exercise in futility.

Everyone has their own issues to deal with. And I would like to let you in on a little secret: because you all came to life in human form, no one person has it "all together." That is why you enlisted to come here—to experience life, work on issues, evolve, and create who you want to be. The others around you are your peers and equals who, like yourself, possess unique attributes and strengths as well as shortcomings. Some of you might be more advanced in one domain, such as love and romance, but deficient in others like career or financial matters. The quality you are lacking may be one someone else is proficient in from whom you can benefit. What you observe in another might be a quality you do not admire, but that trait can be edifying in demonstrating what and how you choose not to be. Treat others as you would want to be treated yourself: it can lead to a greater exchange of energy, talent, ideas, and healing. When you accept and do not prejudge others, you relate on an even platform and tend to give to, share with, and learn from one another more readily and easily. Understanding that you are truly all "one" split up into countless pieces meant to serve and help each other is a huge insight to glean for your healing journey.

The way we view another can either open or block the healing energy that we radiate. When I was in my first month as a medical intern working in the emergency room, a distraught middle-aged woman presented at approximately 4 a.m. shouting, "There are critters in my head, and they are eating my brains!" My senior resident was exhausted, operating on his twentieth consecutive hour of a twenty-four-hour grueling shift. He took one look at her, rolled his eyes in disparagement, and assigned her case to me. He presumed she was not a legitimate medical case and instructed me to do a perfunctory history and physical exam and then quickly send her to the psychiatry service.

However, while I was examining her ears, every time I directed the light of my otoscope inside her ear canal, I saw a black object moving quite wildly. Apparently a cockroach had trespassed and settled there. Whenever the insect stirred, she would start screaming and jumping frantically in uncontrolled fits. But once the cockroach was drowned in mineral oil and flushed out of her middle ear with irrigating fluid, she became a sane and rational woman, thanking me profusely for helping her. She was not mentally deranged; she was a "normal" person expressing heightened fear and anxiety concerning a very real, uncomfortable, and unusual problem. By interacting with her honestly and without prejudgment, I was able to uncover and eradicate the source of her trouble.

Strangers come into your lives with fresh clean canvases. Let them draft their own design and colors onto the surface before you analyze what you perceive. Give them a chance to tell you who they are, where they are coming from, and what they are experiencing and feeling. As they reveal themselves, respond accordingly, but always with honesty, integrity, compassion, respect, and an open mind. When you give others equal standing and your fairmindedness, they tend to bring sincerity and judiciousness to the intercourse. And in the same manner, other people have as great a potential to enhance your sensibilities as you can theirs.

Healing with Wake-up Calls

On occasion there are rare moments in your life when you are rattled or stricken by fraught circumstances that press you to make game-changing decisions or breakthroughs. These often-dramatic events are wake-up calls, and often the more stirring they are, the more significant your growth. The reasons for them are varied. For some it's as if you are stuck at a fork in the road on your life's journey and unable to move forward without a necessary push. For others it may signal a way to get reconnected with your true path. You may have forgotten why you chose to come here, or have become distracted, or have mistakenly traveled off course. Jolting you from your reverie might be all that is needed to move you forward.

In unforeseen and unimaginable ways, it might herald a fortunate reprieve from the brink of disaster, hardship, illness, or physical death not only for your benefit but perhaps also for others.

One such true scenario demonstrates how a wake-up call masquerading as the threat of death offered one young woman important revelations and stirred her to reassess her life and adopt quite an altered attitude. Stacey was a twenty-eight-year-old attorney and wife, pregnant with twins. Of all the many goals in her life, she did not consider motherhood of primary importance. Both the labor and delivery of two healthy boys went rather expeditiously and uneventfully; however, her postpartum period was a different story. A few hours after giving birth, Stacey was experiencing extreme pain in her pelvic and lower abdominal region. She called for the nurse several times and was given some pain medication. The nurse explained to her that discomfort of this nature was to be expected after childbirth as the effects of the epidural were subsiding. Yet the narcotic did not seem to relieve the pain, so she asked the nurse to send for the doctor. Stacey felt that something was critically wrong.

At that point, the nurse looked at Stacey more attentively and noticed that her skin was clammy and her breathing abnormally rapid. She pulled down the bed linens and saw that the sheets were soaked with blood. Stacey's vital signs were unstable; her blood pressure was decreasing, her respiratory rate was accelerating, and her pulse was fast and thready. She was losing blood briskly. Apparently, pieces of her placenta had been inadvertently left inside her uterus, causing her to develop a condition wherein her blood was unable to clot effectively and she was hemorrhaging internally. Stacey was rushed to the operating room where she was given several blood transfusions, her uterus was scraped clean, and she was infused with medicines and fluids respectively to coagulate her blood and rehydrate her.

During this drama, Stacey's heart went into a life-threatening arrhythmia, and the doctors attempted to revive her several times. While all this was occurring, Stacey was experiencing a weightlessness and felt as if she were floating up toward the ceiling and an incredibly warm and soothing light. As the team of doctors and nurses hurriedly and desperately worked to save her life, she was able to view the scenario from above without pain, fear, or worry. A state of total calm and well-being enveloped her.

As she was continuing to gently migrate upward, Stacey suddenly reflected on her two baby boys and the fact that she did not want them to grow up without a mother. Contrary to her previous way of thinking, she now felt a strong maternal instinct to nurture them. At that instant, she perceived herself descending back into her body. The electric paddles shocked her heart to beat in a normal sinus rhythm once again. The medical team sighed with relief. Her bleeding stopped. The twins had their mother back.

You all have a provisional contract with the Universe—goals, ambitions, and improvements that you have come here to achieve. Stacey had not yet fulfilled her contract. It was vitally important that she raise her children and experience the nurturing, protective, and enrapturing bonds of motherhood. Because she had not accomplished all that she had been contracted to do in this lifetime, she chose to return and was whisked from death back into the physical world. The Universe has miraculous and powerful ways of giving you ample opportunities to grow and experience critical events and phenomena for the sake of your highest good. Stacey has stated that if it were not for her two precious sons, she would not have chosen to return to the physical world. She learned to delight in being a mother in ways she never thought she would have. The prospect of death reawakened her to a vital, rewarding, and enriching purpose in her life. She does not regret the choice she made, and now she lives with a newfound knowledge of the joy, serenity, and wisdom that awaits her on the other side. What you can learn from Stacey's story and so many others like hers is that your journey is not over until you have done your best or at least exhausted all attempts to accomplish all commissioned assignments in your lifetime.

Wake-up calls are one way you are prodded to make changes so that healing can occur. The nature and significance of these changes are the topic of the next chapter.

☜ 2 ☞

Change and Healing

The Nature of Change

Change is constant. Accept it or not, it is an unrelenting and ever-present force in your existence that compels you to move forward. The world is not a static environment. As much as you may be content with your lot or feel there is nothing more to be done to improve upon it, powers and influences determining otherwise are set in motion to stir things up and stimulate growth. However you choose to address change—initiate it, seek it, accept it, resist it, elicit it, anticipate it, ignore it, or understand it—some form of call and response is inevitable.

You can either initiate the change you want, or like it or not, change happens to you. Although there are numerous outcomes resulting from change, it is more apt to elicit well-being when you set it in motion than when it is imposed upon you; keep in mind that notable exceptions exist. You may know the change you want to create but not the exact manner to manifest it, and that is alright. Sometimes trial and error is the route you need to follow. Carefully searching for how to enact the right changes plays a crucial part in the healing process.

Change can be difficult to accept. As much as movement in a new direction might help you to evolve in ways beneficial to you, it is natural at times to resist. Change and risk consort with one another. Change upsets the status quo. Its consequences can seem equivocal. In some instances, whether you see your lot as good or bad, at least you know what you have and are aware of what you are dealing with. You tend to hold on to what is established because at one time it may have offered you some sort of happiness, safety, strength, or other satisfaction. The more advantageous those benefits might have once seemed, the more you may want to hold on to the old and defy the new. There is the possibility that events might come into play that may be less favorable than before. Yet the fear that inhabits your mind can sometimes be worse than what actually takes place. Imagination can sometimes take you on extended and unnecessary excursions that feed your fears. The biggest obstacle to change often lies within yourself, and nothing can ultimately shift in your favor until you either accept change or find some way to reconcile and work with it.

As much as the forces of change can lift you up, they can also push you down, and both consequences invariably render some sort of notable impact on you. Life would be so much easier, happier, and more relaxed if the influences of change agreed with you. In those favorable circumstances, by all means *embrace* change, for it is likely to benefit you. When change does not feel right or you resist choosing favorable changes, it can create all sorts of problems—some even detrimental to your health. Its repercussions can invade the mind, the emotions, the body, and even your connection to your soul. Fortunately there are ways to handle unwelcome influences that allow you to move forward with less difficulty.

One of the ways to deal with unwanted change is to first take the time to view it more attentively. Assess whether it might contain any redeeming qualities for you, for others, or for the totality. If you do find any, could they somehow allow you to see change from a different and maybe more accommodating perspective? Flexibility is often an effective way of dealing with these sorts of issues. Can the pros balance or at least attenuate the cons? Would that be a compromise that you could accept and live with? If not, what other options do you have to counter, diminish, or soften change?

At any rate there might be something worthwhile that you can do to endure what is happening more tolerably. By altering your frame of mind—eliciting your own change—you might just have the ability to manage any negative influences. Internal change can sometimes be the most difficult yet the most powerful, brave, efficacious, healthy, and rewarding way of dealing with adversity. In that regard, doing something trumps doing nothing, and the fact that you can formulate a strategic and conscious alteration within yourself might also provide you with a heightened sense of empowerment.

For those of you who are more aware and capable of anticipating change, your forethought has the potential to allow you to act proactively and heighten your chances of an outcome that can be more in line with your particular ideologies and aspirations; otherwise, you might just be resigned to accept what comes. That is fine as long as you are prepared to abide by the consequences.

Sometimes when it might not be expected, the force of change can appear to expand exponentially until its presence is felt on a global level. The magnitude of the combined thoughts, feelings, and actions surrounding it fuel it with such an enormous charge that it would be difficult to halt its propulsive arrival in your world. The epic change may or may not be to your liking, but it still might benefit you to see how and why the overpowering forces of the Universe were responsible for creating it.

No matter what your reactions, know that change is an inevitable and eternal force in life. Whatever changes are present or emerging, search for effective strategies that reflect who you are and who you want to be to deal with them and understand them as best you can.

Searching for Change: The Proper Change to Produce the Preferred Outcome

Change does not always come easily even when you want it desperately. Sometimes the key is in knowing what to revise and how to proceed in order to get your desired results. If you are continually striving unsuccessfully toward your goal, you must modify your approach to achieve your objective. If you find yourself at an impasse, simply halt, take a break, clear your head, reassess matters, back up, and take a different direction. If you are still at a loss as to how to proceed, you might need to take advantage of outside assistance like a friend, relative, mentor, therapist, or clergy. It makes sense: something has to shift in order for you to move forward. Henry Ford said it so eloquently and simply, "If you always do what you've always done, you'll always get what you've always got."

Marty is a handsome yet introverted physical education teacher in his early thirties who kept running into the same impasse when it came to finding a girlfriend.

To understand his problem, we have to go back to his mother. Shortly after his birth, Marty's mother developed mild bouts of mental instability which eventually progressed into long-standing episodes of psychotic behavior. She was unable to be emotionally, physically, and mentally available for him in ways that most mothers are. From the outset, Marty was not able to bond naturally and comfortably with the most important woman in his life. He felt rejected and unloved by her and became angry and resentful toward her.

As an adolescent and adult, he extended his feelings about his mother to members of the opposite sex who he believed were all cold, distant, and repudiating, and yet he yearned to be loved by them. He was sending out conflicting messages to the Universe: "Hey ladies, you are all unkind, distant, and hurtful, but I do want to find love and be loved by you." He tried meeting women in bars, at social gatherings, dances, and nightclubs, and on the internet to no avail. It was not surprising that the women he encountered all confirmed his image of them. The energy he transmitted, he also attracted. What an uncomfortable dilemma in which to be trapped! What Marty needed to do was to heal the hurt and pain emanating from his traumatic past and dissociate his unfavorable experiences and perceptions of his mother with how he collectively viewed the female gender. It was imperative that he modify the signals he was broadcasting and instead declare and acknowledge: "Hey ladies, I know that the world is full of wonderful, kind, loving, warm, and nurturing members of your gender, and I am ready, willing, and able to experience a relationship based on those views."

Marty is a work in progress. He is seeing a therapist and working on his issues. Hopefully one day this emotionally scarred young man will be able to heal by changing his perspective and sharing the love he so desperately desires with the right woman.

Accepting Change: The Universe Creates Change for a Reason

Sometimes the changes that occur in your life are not what you would have chosen for yourself at that moment, but in retrospect, they are exactly what you needed. To return to one of my favorite maxims: you may plan your life, but every so often accidents or inconveniences control it. These occurrences are essentially the wise forces of the Universe pushing you in directions you may feel compelled to follow. To understand why, it is important to look at the big picture—the forest and not the trees. When you see all the pieces of the puzzle and know all the events in a story, your understanding becomes clearer and the complete view seems to make more sense. You might not have been content with all the steps leading up to the outcome, but you may eventually realize that each step was particularly crucial to attain the net result.

Such an inescapable adoption of change is demonstrated by events that happened to an acquaintance of mine. One summer, Mallory was planning and looking forward to backpacking in Europe. Unfortunately, shortly before she was to depart, she stumbled, broke her ankle, and her lower extremity was partially immobilized in a plaster cast. To her dismay, she had to abruptly change her plans. She canceled her trip and stayed home with her parents that summer.

She and her father did not share a close or cordial relationship. He had just retired. The forces that be could not have chosen a more compellingly awkward yet opportune time for them to be together. Unexpectedly, while both were working on the garden, they bonded in ways they had been unable to before and reached a new level of awareness, appreciation, and affection for each other. Another unfortunate and unexpected event occurred toward the end of that summer: Mallory's father passed from a heart attack. Although Mallory initially had been disappointed to stay home with her parents, she soon realized how blessed she had been that such an inauspicious turn of events forced her to spend meaningful and valuable time with her dad. She felt that the Universe, in its mysterious and camouflaged manner, had given her an extra six-week bonus period to mend her differences, reach an understanding, and become reacquainted with her father. As their garden grew more rich and beautiful, so did their connection. At his funeral, she was able to bid him farewell without the regret of an unresolved relationship.

No matter how you look at it, if you can allow it, change sometimes has the potential to transport you to a much more evolved and enlightened station whether or not you would have consciously chosen that path. Your soul, that part of you that watches over you and guides you in the best direction, knows what is ultimately optimal for you, like it or not. Trust it. You might as well enjoy the journey since it is all taking place in your best interest and expressly for you. When circumstances have you feeling stuck, tense, and confused, it can sometimes be a comforting and liberating thought that what is happening is simply serving your highest good as orchestrated by more highly evolved, healing, and wise forces.

Resisting Change in an Unhealthy Way

Stubborn resistance to change can sometimes lead to disease or death. In the same way that certain businesses cannot flourish if they do not align themselves with beneficial emerging large-scale trends, your bodies cannot thrive if you oppose sound and rational adjustment and compromise. Some people deal unreasonably with disruption, and they pay a heavy price for it. They may feel entitled to their established conditions. They may feel like a victim and blame others for unwelcome disturbance. They may hold on to feelings like anger, fear, bitterness, hate, and resentment. They may not bounce back easily from interference. They may not have learned to be more flexible or proactive when change occurs. They may lack the awareness to look inside for answers and to see how they might be responsible for their circumstances and what they can do to better forge ahead. They may tend to become more infirm than people who react shrewdly and resourcefully to unwelcome influences.

Here is one extreme example of how resisting change caused one couple to develop serious afflictions. Lorraine and Daniel were a well-to-do retired couple who many years earlier had set up a trust fund for their daughter, Anne. A very close friend of Daniel's, Bob, was a banker who offered to set up the fund. Years passed, and Anne married a lawyer named William and they had two daughters. One day, William was going over the trust fund documents and discovered grave technical flaws. Apparently these errors were so serious that there was concern for their legality. In order to correct matters, William initiated judicial action against the bank and, indirectly, Bob. Daniel and Lorraine were shocked. They were embarrassed and ashamed that their daughter and son-in-law were suing one of their good friends. They tried to persuade Anne and William to settle this matter in a more private and civil way to no avail; the two were determined to forge ahead full throttle with the lawsuit.

The verdict revealed the bank to be at fault. Anne and William received a monetary sum in compensation. The bank was fined for its wrongdoings, and Bob suffered some disciplinary action. Unfortunately as a result of the whole ordeal, Lorraine and Daniel were on cold and distant terms with Bob, Anne, and William. Daniel was intent on placing blame with his son-in-law and daughter for the whole fiasco. He was angry that they did not try to resolve the matter out of court. He demanded that Lorraine do as he had decided to do and sever all relations with their daughter and son-in-law. She apprehensively conceded. Now they were also estranged from their grandchildren. As time passed, Lorraine and Daniel lived in silence with their anguish. Whenever their friends discussed their own children or grandchildren, their hearts would freeze with pangs of loss and shame while their bitterness simmered.

Lorraine was extremely distraught and unsettled over this decision, and she vacillated between making amends and maintaining the separation. Her physical health also suffered. Over time she lost her appetite and developed intestinal pain, back pain, eczema, shingles, neuralgia, migraine headaches, insomnia, and depression. She frequented a slew of doctors and therapists, but no treatment comforted her. She ached with a yearning to be with her daughter and granddaughters again. She could not comprehend how Daniel could purge them from his life so completely. She desperately wanted to find a different way to be that would alleviate her mental anguish.

She pleaded with him to reconsider. He told her that if she ever attempted to reunite with them, their marriage would be over. Torn between her husband and her offspring, she felt like a tortured soul. Soon she stopped going out in public. Her body became emaciated. As time passed, she became bedridden, feeble, a mere wisp of the woman she once was, and ultimately succumbed to her own tormented emotions.

Their saga illustrates a dramatic case of not being able to reevaluate a position and make changes. Whether their daughter was right or wrong is inconsequential. Lorraine's troubled feelings not only denied her of her ability to forgive but also drained her life's energy. The Universe forgives all and wants you to learn to forgive each other. Lorraine did make a decision to renounce her daughter, but intentions can be altered. No determination of that nature is set in stone. Her physical body was sending her numerous messages to redirect her from her misery, but she was marooned in her own tormented psyche and unfortunately not open to its wisdom. And then there was Daniel's threat. That certainly added angst to her already harrowed heart. She had to choose to either stand by her man or by her child—two agonizingly punishing options. Who is to say what Daniel would have actually done had she forgiven Anne. Sometimes actions speak an entirely different language than words. In the end it was all too much for her system to handle—torn between holding on to her anguish, acrimony, and ambivalence versus relenting and forgiving.

Even after his wife's death, Daniel could not allow himself to release his fury. Gradually he began to suffer mental lapses. Containing his rage drained so much energy from his psyche that it was easier for him to detach from reality. At the time of this writing, it is still not too late for Daniel to change. It could prove to be the toughest and most courageous step in his life—and also the most healing one.

Lorraine and Daniel's case demonstrates that despite great pain, some individuals hold on to the situations that they have themselves created and lack the fortitude and awareness to make vital propitious changes. They are so mired in anger, pride, obstinacy, fear, or torment that they cannot see or find a more favorable way out. It is difficult to imagine why someone would live with such anguish when other options are available, but many do. Unfortunately some people pay a harsh price for resisting change.

Eliciting Internal Change

The following prayer regarding change by Reinhold Niebuhr—commonly referred to as the Serenity Prayer—can be a great resource for obtaining peace and resolution in difficult circumstances:

> God, please grant me the serenity
> to accept the things I cannot change,
> the courage to change the things I can
> and wisdom to know the difference.

It is a profound insight when you realize that you have little or no power to affect what is outside your control but rather a great deal more power to adjust your own perspective or plans. Sometimes one of the toughest lessons and strongest displays of determination and grit resides in finding out that the answer to your plight lies in bringing about change within yourself and not in wittingly modifying any external condition or force. That is not to say that your ability to influence others is trifling and ineffectual, but if you do reach an impasse, you have more command over yourself than you do over anyone else. What's more, what feels right to you may not seem the same to another. When you alter your mind in order to move forward when it is not possible to sway someone else to think or act as you do, you are the one who has evolved and elevated your consciousness in a grand way. Internal change is one of the most powerful and venerable forms of transformation. The following story may help to clarify why.

Betsey is a sixty-eight-year-old woman who grew up in the East Village of Manhattan. Her family was not wealthy, but they were comfortable. When she was in her mid-teens, she socialized with a few girls from the surrounding neighborhoods. One of those girls was her second cousin Delia, who was from the more affluent neighborhood of Gramercy Park. One afternoon the girls decided that they wanted to see a Broadway matinee. Betsey was excited because she did not often go to the theater. While they were discussing which play they wanted to see and the logistics of getting to the show, Delia burst out with the comment, "I wonder whether Betsey will be able to afford a ticket!" Up to that point, Betsey had been enjoying herself and did not feel any different than the other girls. She was stunned and embarrassed by her cousin's remark. Now she pondered whether she was worthy enough to be in their company.

After that, Betsey distanced herself from Delia. It was not an entirely conscious decision. She lacked self-confidence and was particularly more aware of that fact and more uncomfortable when she was in Delia's presence. Her mother would often ask her, "Why don't you get together with your cousin Delia? She is such a nice girl." Years passed, Betsey got married, moved to the Upper West Side, had children, and unfortunately became a widow. She never forgot her mother's remarks to befriend Delia and deep inside she still felt bad that she could not develop a closer bond with her cousin. To go through the discomfort and humiliation of reconnecting with Delia was certainly not a priority; besides, she had other friends, and she remembered how fraught with shame she had felt in Delia's company.

Then one day she unexpectedly ran into Delia who had just joined her ethnic dancing class. Betsey loved the class. She had been taking it for about a year. The instructor Donny was dynamic, charismatic, and upbeat, and he made the steps easy to follow and fun to learn. The other students were convivial, appealing, cheerful, and broad-minded and seemed to resonate to the same energy as the teacher. Many, including Betsey, socialized with one another outside of class and found they had other interests in common.

At first Betsey was delighted to see Delia at the class. She took it upon herself to introduce her to her friends and show her the ropes. She never expected her cousin to turn them into a noose. Delia was quick to make judgments. "Isn't Donny one of *those* types of people?" Betsey knew what Delia was intimating. "Yes," she responded, "Donny is gay, and he is a wonderful dance instructor and a beautiful person!" Later after class, Delia asked Betsey which temple she belonged to and how often she attended services. Betsey had a strong belief in God and considered herself to be more spiritual than devoutly religious. She told her cousin that she was a member of a Reform synagogue and went to shul on the High Holy Days. To that her cousin retorted, "So you are one of *those* types of Jews!" Suddenly, Betsey had an epiphany and realized exactly why she had distanced herself from Delia: she never really liked her cousin. Delia had been judgmental, narrow-minded, pompous, and elitist as a teenager and stayed pretty much the same as an adult. Delia had not changed, but Betsey had. Betsey had learned to like herself and be confident in who she is. She no longer considered herself unworthy of Delia but instead felt sorry that her cousin was alienating and depriving herself of many wonderful people and opportunities. After so many years, she was finally able to see both herself and her cousin in a clearer light. There was good reason she had not sought out Delia's company despite her mother's nudging. Betsey no longer felt compelled to befriend Delia, who, not surprisingly, decided to drop the dance class.

Betsey had no control over Delia's attitude and behavior, but she did have the insight, inner strength, and courage to acknowledge and embrace her own ways of thinking. Delia's disposition demonstrated to Betsey the qualities she did not desire to espouse and ultimately made her realize that she is self-confident and does like who she is. It took her over fifty years to understand exactly why she did not want to spend more time with her cousin and why that was perfectly alright. She had made a monumental shift in consciousness.

Anticipating and Ignoring Change: A Tale of Two Sisters

You are all responsible for creating change in your lives. Was the man trapped in the burning building actually a victim? What if it were discovered that he had procrastinated fixing a loose electrical wire in a light switch in the kitchen? Had he been proactive, the blaze might have been avoided. Anticipation is a key element in how you can alter the outcome of your lives. Many wait until lightning strikes to bring about change. Look at the example of the obese person who suffers a heart attack or the smoker who is diagnosed with chronic obstructive pulmonary disease. Whether you know it or not, you create your destiny, but it is not always as apparent as in these examples. Circumstances are set up by your soul to act as catalysts to spur you forward in your evolution. When there is hope of and opportunity for growth, you are bestowed with additional chances to amend your course. For instance, the recovered cardiac patient may choose to modify his lifestyle by adopting healthy habits related to diet, physical activity, workload, stress levels, recreation, and attitudes.

The following illustration portrays the different ways two women anticipated change and the ensuing effects on their facial skin. Sara and Diana are two sisters in their mid-thirties. Although they look alike and share a propensity for cystic acne, they are worlds apart when it comes to dealing with change. Sara, two years younger with an MBA, worked as a vice president for an international bank. It was the position she had always wanted, but after almost two years she realized that it no longer excited or fulfilled her. She now found it insipid and tedious. Her facial acne was active with pustules and inflamed cysts. Her physical body was sending her a message via her skin that something in her life was not right. The attractive six-figure income and generous benefits package of a pension, health insurance coverage, four weeks of vacation a year, and an annual bonus no longer seemed important compared to job satisfaction. She longed to be more passionate about her work. Television production seemed enticing. Having had no experience in that area, she decided to volunteer her services a few evenings a week and one day each weekend at a local television network while she continued to work at the bank.

Transformed from an esteemed banking executive to a volunteer gofer at a television studio, she never complained. She felt fortunate and excited to be there and absorb as much information and experience as she could. She was a fast learner. When a key production assistant called in sick one day on an important assignment, Sara was asked to fill in. Not only was she glad to help out in a pinch, but she also offered some valuable suggestions so that the work moved more smoothly and efficiently. After that lucky break, she was offered a full-time position. She gave notice at the bank. Her family and some of her friends and associates thought that she had gone batty, leaving a desirable, distinguished, and highly paid position in finance for an entry-level job as a production assistant at a music television station, but she was thrilled. Without any other changes in her skin care regimen, her acne began to clear. In every project that she handled she excelled, and the executives at the station took notice. She was advancing expeditiously in her new career. Eventually she was promoted to a position of associate producer.

Diana, the older sister, also with an MBA, was a director of marketing for an international tobacco company with offices in New York. Unfortunately she clung to a false sense of security in her professional life and did not effectively evaluate her situation and anticipate change. The economy was on a downswing, and the tobacco industry was no longer working with the same generous budget as it had in the past. With a growing health-conscious environment, her company was venturing to diversify its base beyond cigarettes and cigars while at the same time struggling to increase profits. She decided to ignore any contemplated notices of cutbacks as she did not feel they were likely or, if they did occur, they would not possibly affect her. After all, she had been with the company for a long time and had moved up the ranks to become a high-level executive. Finally, shortly after the fall of the World Trade Center, the board of directors decided to relocate the New York offices to Virginia to save on expenses. The deal offered to employees was that anyone who wanted to transfer south was welcome, and anyone not interested would be entitled to a severance package based upon their length of time with the firm. Over the next year, pink slips were being sent out in a series of waves for those who elected not to transfer.

Diana chose not to relocate. She felt that she had more than enough time to find a comparable position with another New York firm. She deemed that she would be assigned to the last wave of employees to be let go because she regarded her area of expertise as extremely valuable to the operations of her department. Instead, she was among the first to get a pink slip. She was stunned. She had not accurately anticipated change. Furthermore, she had trouble securing employment. Not surprisingly her facial acne erupted. The period spent out of work did give Diana an opportunity to reflect on her circumstances and, how if another similar situation should arise, she could anticipate and prepare for change more effectively.

Two tales. Two sisters. One proactive and the other reactive. One creating and embracing new opportunities, the other clinging to ineffectual modes of thinking. One clearing up her skin disorder, the other suffering more prolonged outbreaks. The two sisters could not be more disparate in their attitudes toward change. This story reveals how it can be prudent to anticipate, confront, and welcome change and how the physical body can often let you know when you have not.

Understanding Change on a Global Scale

The Universe has a way of manifesting change for your highest good, even if it occasionally creates disguised opportunities. Because global transformation is such a huge, complicated endeavor, it often sneaks up mysteriously but with a mighty impact. You might not see it coming, but when it makes its mark, it is so powerful that you cannot ignore or refute it. Like it or not, everything happens for a reason. A tragic or dramatic event is sometimes needed to bring about some unexpected progressive consequences. It is prudent to view it from a broader perspective rather than from its individual parts to appreciate the value of the change.

Organ donation was a rare practice in Italy until the mid to late 1990s when a tragic incident awakened the consciousness of its people. An Anglo-American family was on holiday making their way south by car along the western coast of Italy. One night on a vacant strip of highway, a group of armed bandits fired their guns at the family's car. Nicholas Green, a seven-year-old boy asleep in the back seat, was hit in the head by a stray bullet. Rushed to the hospital, his body was alive and functioning with the aid of life support equipment, but his brain could not be saved. His parents courageously made a painful decision to release his soul from his body. Before doing so, they offered many of his viable and desperately needed organs to those suffering with degenerating physical parts. His corneas, kidneys, pancreas, liver, and heart were of no use to him anymore.

The senseless shooting of this young boy was no longer without purpose. Even after his death, his life had significant merit. Not only did he restore life and health to several afflicted individuals via his organs, but the unfortunate events that transpired awakened the country to the need for and importance of organ donation and transplantation—at the time an uncommon medical practice which had been resisted to a large extent. The local and international media had broadcast throughout Italy and the world the uplifting and positive side of this tragedy. Nicholas's death and sacrifice helped expand the consciousness of people everywhere—greatly benefiting society. His father always felt strongly that Nicholas was a mighty force who one day would do great deeds. The Universe's plan disguised as misfortune brought about a positive impact to humanity that might not have materialized as receptively and readily had the circumstances not been as dramatic as they were.

The next chapter deals with the topic of spiritual guidance. Like change, it is another mighty force with both internal and external ramifications and holds amazing capabilities to direct you in ways that serve your highest good. It is one of the four major components of your being that influences your health.

≈ 3 ≈

Healing on a Spiritual Level

The Nature of Spiritual Guidance

Of all the different levels of your being on which you heal—physical, emotional, mental, and spiritual—the last one is probably the most advanced and complex. There are two reasons why I am choosing to begin with it. First, by understanding the intricacies and functions of your spiritual essence, you may find it easier to understand the other three. Second, spiritual guidance plays a vital role in facilitating the other three levels in moving forward in the best possible way. It is usually the last of the four healing dimensions to be recognized and developed. In some cultures, particularly in Western and technologically advanced ones, it is not accorded as high a regard as the others. More emphasis is placed on physicality, cognition, and feelings—and usually in that order. Most of you do not develop a true sense of spirituality until you have evolved either by spending some quality time in the deep caverns of your psyche or by experiencing a significant crisis of some sort. Dealing with a major hardship can often act as a catalyst to initiate or reaffirm a connection with your spiritual faculties. However, there is no typical age in which this phase ripens. Some individuals are spiritually aware early on, while some senior citizens are clueless. The very fact that you are reading about this topic now means that your higher self or soul has deemed you ready to explore this part of your being.

One common mistake is to confuse spirituality and religion. A person may be devout with regard to a chosen faith but may or may not be spiritual. Many of the statutes and customs of organized religion are man-made. The proper foods to ingest and views concerning marriage, sex, and attire are just a few examples. In no way do I claim to judge or critique anyone's beliefs, but I do feel that spirituality transcends all religions. It is universal, and its essence abides irrespective of religious affiliation. Belief in a higher nonphysical and more enlightened power or source of guidance or whatever one considers as such is a prerequisite, but it is the way you conduct your life, regardless of your beliefs or affiliations, that is of prime importance. A sense of the innate and authentic principles of fairness, love, forgiveness, honesty, compassion, and faith are some of the qualities that define the character of a spiritually enlightened being.

Signs from the Universe

All happenings—whether seemingly ordinary or not— have a deeper meaning and source than they appear to on the surface. Everything in your world is orchestrated for a reason, and it is the quest of the spiritually enlightened to ponder why, search for answers, and find resolution. If you are not aware, curious, and open to search for guidance and messages, they will most likely pass you by.

Underlying all the activity, congestion, and confusion in your lives are disguised events and signs acting as catalysts to spur you to growth and transformation. Seek and you shall find the answers, but if you never search, no counsel may be evident. Signs guiding you toward the light are planted all around you, but the Universe does not operate by spoon-feeding. When you are willing, ready, and able to be receptive to fresh possibilities and look beyond the borders of your mundane existence, your comfort zone, and your purported certitude, an incredible illuminating reality awaits you.

When seeking guidance through signs, it is alright—and indeed recommended—that you consciously ask for help and await a message. Acting this way not only initiates the process and facilitates the dispatch, but also alerts you to be more receptive of a reply. The response may not always arrive as clearly, expeditiously, or directly as you would like, but it is sure to appear in some form. The pertinent message may be as subtle as lyrics from a song you hear on the radio or the title of a book that mysteriously falls off your shelf or as blatant and direct as your spouse repeating the identical words of advice that you just heard from your therapist hours earlier. The key point is to prime your consciousness not only to be amenable to asking for help and direction, but also disposed to receive, acknowledge, and interpret the answers no matter how faint or marked they may be.

Some people are oblivious or even resistant to signs of help or warning; nevertheless, they are still as welcome to the beneficial intimations from the Universe as those seeking aid. Their hints just might need to carry more zing for them to get the message. Also when the pronouncement is of a more pressing or significant nature, the signs tend to be more dramatic, intense, or unremitting.

Jessie is a chronic two-pack-a-day cigarette smoker. His family has been on his case to quit his pernicious habit for a long while but to no avail. Although he has ignored his worsening symptoms of a relentless cough and shortness of breath as well as the various annoying anti-smoking remedies incessantly advertised on his computer, television, and in magazines, he could not disregard the ultimate and most alarming message from the Universe when he learned that his best smoking buddy had been diagnosed with advanced lung cancer. The Universe persists with more threatening signs until some purposeful response registers.

So if you happen to be in need of some higher guidance, whether or not you wittingly ask, be prudent and mindful of any covert or conspicuous signs that may appear.

Humor as a Way for Spirit to Convey a Message

The spiritual realm is no different than the physical world when it comes to wit to perk your attention. Sometimes you need a dose of comic relief to break out of the doldrums or heal a saddened psyche. However, the spirit world has the added advantage of perfect timing in the most surprising of ways and with a sixth sense for how you will react. The following is a surprising real-life scenario demonstrating this fanciful humor.

Jennifer is a broad-minded and evolved young woman of twenty-nine who had a very close bond with her grandfather. Even though she lived in New York and he lived in Florida, they would communicate often over the phone. One of the many qualities that she loved and admired about him was his offbeat and quirky sense of humor. He could make her laugh at the most inopportune times and on the slightest pretext.

Suddenly and unexpectedly, Jennifer's grandfather passed away from a heart attack. She was devastated and had not had the chance to say goodbye. She longed and prayed for some sign from him that he was alright. Since most of his relatives and his final resting place were in New York, his body was shipped north for memorial services and burial. On the day of the funeral, Jennifer's cell phone had run out of power since in her mourning she had forgotten to charge it. When family and friends arrived at the grave site to convey their final prayers and sentiments, the casket accidentally fell and opened before the gravediggers had lowered it into the ground. Much to everyone's dismay, the corpse was not Jennifer's grandfather. Most of the guests were either mortified or outraged, but not Jennifer. She looked up at the sky and smiled, knowing full well that it was her grandfather's warped sense of humor that had orchestrated this mix-up. And as if that were not enough to confirm her suspicions, during all the commotion her cell phone inexplicably rang. When she answered it, there was silence, yet the caller ID displayed her grandfather's telephone number. Jennifer was the only one laughing aloud in the cemetery because she had received an undeniable sign in her grandfather's signature waggish style that he was indeed okay.

Jennifer possesses the spiritual awareness that there is so much more than what she perceives within the confines of her physical reality. For those who are unable to conceptualize a transcendental dimension, such messages are unavailable. You can never genuinely perceive what you are not open to receive. If you unlock your minds to assimilate all the extraordinary possibilities that exist in the world, it might just astound you to discover how vast, wondrous, and truly funny they can be.

Understanding Spiritual Guidance

In order to understand spiritual guidance, it is important to simplify this abstract and complex subject. You may ask, "What is the specific source of this guidance and why should I trust it? I cannot see, hear, or touch this counsel in any form I am accustomed to." Skepticism is just as much an admirable quality as broad-mindedness. As with any unfamiliar idea you are introduced to, you should muster your curiosity as well as your scrutiny to assess what it is all about and whether it is worth the risk to explore further. But for those who never elect to take that chance, there is surely nothing to be gained.

One of the prime aspects of spiritual guidance either from your soul or spirit guide is that it is kind, nurturing, and unconditionally loving. It seeks to serve your highest good. Each being has a divine plan or purpose mapped out by the soul, and it is your soul or your spirit guide's great joy to steer you in that direction. If you wander off course, it is their aim to send you clues to help get you back on track.

In order to better comprehend this topic, it is important to clarify the meaning of the soul and the spirit guide. Your soul, also known as higher self or knowing self, is *your* spirit, quite distinct from your spirit guide. It is your ethereal essence that has been and will be with you forever. It contains all your thoughts, memories, dreams, wishes, feelings, and experiences from every lifetime and the intervals between them. It is the life force assigned to and accompanying the physical body at the commencement of your incarnation and released from it at death.

One of its key objectives while connected to your physical form is to experience, grow, and create in the grandest version of the greatest vision of who you are. It has access to your life purpose, your talents, and your undeveloped potential and helps you to comprehend who you are and discover who you want to be. Your soul tries to communicate with you, guide you, and even create circumstances or opportunities that can help you to evolve. Some of you are more adept at interacting with your soul. The soul inherently exists in a nonphysical dimension, yet it is enriched by its intangible bond with the body, just as most birds innately inhabit the sky—akin to the soul's natural home in the invisible spiritual space known as the aether—but do occasionally wander on land and sea—akin to the soul's temporary visitation in the physical realm associated with a body. On the other hand, your spirit guide is like a wise advisor who is distinctly and carefully chosen to counsel you concerning your specific objectives and interests as well as a vast array of other issues in your lifetime with your soul acting as an intermediary. Your spirit guide, just as your soul, is always present and often attempts to send you advice whether or not you are aware. Once you establish reliable and conscious communication with either of these entities, the relationship can be an incredibly rewarding source of wisdom, inspiration, and opportunities for growth. The scope of guidance of the soul and spirit guide overlaps and can also be different, but neither is wrong. It would be difficult to differentiate and delineate all their myriad functions; however, it would be accurate to say that the spirit guide provides additional specialized content aligned with your particular worldly interests while the soul focuses on actualizing and enhancing your inherent purpose.

Spirit (short for spirit guide) is like a combination of a best friend, nurturing parent, guidance counselor, and wise mentor whose connection to you is available at all times—you can call upon him, her, or it at any moment of the day or night to counsel, console, teach, heal, or help you. Spirit has no gender in the way you might perceive it but does share characteristics that may be aligned with one sex more than the other. It might have more knowledge of electronics or romance, qualities your society equates to be more masculine or feminine, respectively. Spirit, also known as your Higher Wisdom, is extremely judicious, intelligent, and nonjudgmental and would never deny you assistance unless, of course, the help that you request would not serve your highest good. Spirit is like a liaison between you and the Universe. You actually attract spirit guides whose interests would most benefit you or whose areas of expertise mesh most with your own. Some of you have more than one spirit guide or have acquired other guides throughout your lifetime as you have matured or evolved in directions that make you more amenable to enlightenment from different types of teachers. What you might have once needed from a particular spirit guide no longer serves you in just the same way as you no longer need the assistance of your college advisor after you graduate university. There are critical junctures in your life when you might be ripe for a new or different type of mentor more in tune with your changing interests and evolution.

Some, but not all spirit guides, have previously been on the physical plane as human beings. Those who were have mastered the necessary tasks and requirements to "graduate" or move ahead are eligible to serve you from a higher dimension. Not every soul who departs your dimension elects or is qualified to be a spirit guide. It is similar to teaching assistants in college. They too once started out as novice students, but because of a combination of their strong and evolved character, their commitment to excellence in their areas of expertise, and their prime interpersonal and teaching skills, they were chosen by the professor to advise other students. Other spirit guides who have never experienced a lifetime on the earthly plane come from much more advanced dimensions of the cosmos and have elected with great joy and privilege to aid and enrich you with their expertise and wisdom.

Some of you are more aligned and in touch with Spirit, while others have had glimpses through dreams, signs, or other intuitive dispatches. Regardless of how connected you may be, there is always the possibility to formally initiate, reestablish, or strengthen your bond. Your spirit guides are always able, willing, and more than ready to serve. It is merely up to you to acknowledge your Higher Wisdom and formally begin the relationship. Prior to that point, Spirit has always been with you sending you messages that you either received unawares or that you totally disregarded. It is akin to entering a party lounge full of people drinking and socializing while a radio is playing popular music at a modest decibel level in the background. Your ears hear the radio, yet your consciousness may not actually focus upon and register the music and lyrics unless you make a concerted effort to tune out the excess ambient stimuli in the room. Learning to communicate with Spirit is like training your consciousness to direct your attention this way.

Young children are generally more able to see, hear, feel, and communicate with the spiritual world. They are closer to that realm than adults since they only recently arrived here from there during their gestational period. After birth, infants go through a trying transitional period when they slowly detach from their ethereal reality in order to adjust to the physical one. Little ones typically and quite naturally may interact with stuffed animals, dolls, blankets, or imaginary friends as one way to communicate with the spirit world. However, many of you live in a culture that does not value or acknowledge connecting with the spirit realm. Either directly or indirectly, as you mature, many of you surrender to the influences of conditioning and assimilate society's mores. Yet some of you defy convention and either adapt by practicing your beliefs openly or on the side or at some later period in your lives spawn enough pluck to reconnect.

The following account demonstrates how receptive children can be to the influences of the spirit world. Ina lost her father to a brain tumor when she was eleven years old. The impact was so great she fell into a deep depression. For about a year she ate poorly, slept restlessly, hardly talked or smiled, and had difficulty in school. Although she eventually moved on, even as an adult the loss of her father still left a powerful emotional scar on her psyche. She often spoke of him with both deep love and sadness.

Fast-forward to her late twenties. Ina had married and was the mother of a two-year-old boy named Darrel. Darrel was an active, happy, and talkative little boy who did not like to sleep. After Ina and her husband would tuck Darrel into bed, they would hear him talking periodically throughout the night. Sometimes Ina would open the door to his room and peek inside and observe Darrel quite contentedly chatting away in gibberish sounds that she did not understand. On a few occasions she queried

Darrel as to what he was talking about. He would always tell her that he was conversing with a nice man. "He is my friend, mommy. He likes me, and he helps me." Ina had just accepted that explanation as typical of the "imaginary friends" some young children have. She acknowledged Darrel's discussions, but she did not encourage or challenge them.

When Darrel was about four years old, Ina's mother came to visit from the Dominican Republic. She brought a photo album with her to share some memories. One evening she was sitting on the couch with Ina and Darrel looking over old photographs. Suddenly Darrel screamed, "Mommy, Mommy, that is my friend. There he is!" as he pointed to a photograph of Ina's father. Darrel had never seen a picture of his grandfather before, but he knew the man who visited him each night and was sure that he was the man in the picture. There were photographs of many people both alive and deceased in the album: cousins, uncles, aunts, grandparents, and friends. The only one he recognized was his maternal grandfather.

Ina became emotional. She looked at her son and then viewed the picture of her dad, and tears started to roll down her cheeks. She was overjoyed because she now perceived that her father was still around her. Although she had not been aware of his spiritual presence before, she now knew that he came to her in spirit through her son. It took approximately nineteen years for her to receive a sign from her father. Her loss was not as raw anymore. Shortly after the discovery of the identity of Darrel's imaginary friend, the visits ceased. Darrel no longer talked about his friend. Perhaps the father's main objective, besides getting to know and support his grandson, was to give his daughter something that she had never been able to feel after his abrupt physical death—the peace of mind and knowledge that he was alright and still watching over her.

Although it is beyond the intended purview of this book to elaborate on the visitations and communications of departed souls of loved ones, friends, and relatives as these energies can be of a much more diverse nature, many people do experience such phenomena. Their presence can be extremely valuable especially to those like Ina who are still quite unsettled from someone's passing. Although many revisiting souls can and do deliver great comfort, assistance, and information to those on the physical plane, others, usually those with no prior connection to you, long to come back yet may lack the appropriate skills or high-level guidance. You may inquire of all communicating spirits if they are of a high level or if they are from the "light," for they are not permitted to deceive you. If for any reason you detect that the energy of a guide or spirit does not feel right, you can always sever the connection by simply requesting that they depart your presence.

Another way to think of your connection to your spirit guide or soul is like having a link to an intuitive or sixth sense. Channeling Spirit is an aptitude which you all possess and have the ability to develop. Think of this ability or sense as a muscle. The more you exercise it, the more proficient it becomes and the more deftly it performs. Like any skill, for some it comes more easily and naturally than for others. Take basketball for instance; not everyone can play as expertly as Michael Jordan, but you can all learn the game. The point is that you are all capable of developing some level of proficiency.

Each of you attracts spirit guides whose expertise matches your own interests. Just as you are inherently drawn to a specific career or hobby such as computer technology, education, acupuncture, painting, singing, soccer, etc., each spirit guide is intrinsically highly skilled and knowledgeable in their own particular field of interest. You tend to devote more attention to whatever your interests and aspirations are and inevitably attract specific spirit guides who can support you in those areas.

In order to avoid confusion and since, to a large degree, there is much overlap and not a significant difference in what they provide you, going forward in this book, the soul and the spirit guide will hereby be addressed collectively as "Spirit" unless otherwise noted. If you are not clear and want to know with whom you are communicating, simply ask. As with any relationship over time, you will eventually become proficient in recognizing the source of your communications.

How to Seek Spiritual Guidance

There is not just one surefire and easy streamlined way to connect with Spirit. Does one simply look up to the sky and announce, "Hey, Spirit, I am now ready to meet you!"? Although there are innumerable ways to get acquainted, that certainly would not be a bad start. Meeting Spirit is a process, and it materializes differently for each of you. It is much like finding a mate. Some of you encounter that person early in life, others late, some by actively searching, others by happenstance, some at a dance, others at school or work, etc. The possibilities and permutations are practically endless. One prerequisite is to be open, curious, or desirous of forming such a bond. You certainly would not attract a mate if you do not send out appropriate signals and energy. The same holds true with regard to attracting Spirit.

Another important condition for meeting Spirit is to clear your mind of annoying internal buzz and chatter. Spirit would be drowned out if the amount of stimulation in the mind is loud and chaotic. A serene and stable environment is a more appropriate and conducive setting to channel. One helpful way to prepare the atmosphere for your Higher Wisdom to enter is to practice meditation. What this does, besides generally helping to bring about a healthier physical, mental, emotional, and spiritual state, is to train the mind to be more aware, serene, focused, and refreshed. It is difficult to make healthy new acquaintances at times in life when confusion, chaos, and/or lethargy prevail. Meditation provides a means to calm your mind and raise your vibration so that you can make your frequency more compatible with the higher-frequency energy field of Spirit and thus create a more optimal setting to interface.

The last key element necessary to channel Spirit is to simply attempt making a connection, which will be presented later in this chapter in a meditative exercise. The more you make efforts to bond, the closer you can get to establishing a clear channel of communication. Practice makes perfect, so do not be disappointed if contact is not made on the initial try. It is much like operating a ham radio. To tune in to the correct frequency and then wait patiently for someone out there to listen and respond may take some time, patience, practice, and perseverance. You need to learn to raise your vibration to a higher frequency just as much as Spirit must work to lower theirs so that your two energies can connect. And when you do finally make contact, transmission may at first be weak and subtle, but as in most disciplines, the more you practice, the better and more proficient you become at achieving your goal, and in this case, the stronger the channel connection becomes.

Do not be surprised if the nature of the communication is different than you expect. The messages come in many forms. For some they may be auditory, just like hearing someone talk or listening to a song on the radio, only inside your head. When in the presence of others, no one else seems to be aware of what you are hearing. This first method of spiritual transmission is referred to as *clairaudience*. The main difference between clairaudience and the voices described in individuals suffering from psychosis is that in the former the nuance of the message is uplifting, supportive, loving, and kind, whereas those of the latter might have cynical, abusive, or pejorative overtones.

Communiqués can also sometimes be presented visually, like watching a silent film, seeing a photograph, or viewing a dream. In ways that are uniquely intelligible to the one receiving the visual perception, these visions may offer understanding or insight into a situation or question that warrants guidance. This way of receiving knowledge is known as *clairvoyance*.

Channeled messages may also come to you as moments of profound insight like an epiphany, a thought that you know to be incontrovertibly true without having received any information regarding it in a traditional manner. This knowledge may pertain to people, places, things, or situations. One example might be knowing that your sister-in-law is pregnant before she has started to show signs and maybe even before she is aware of it. Sometimes unexplained emotions like joy or dread may suddenly come upon you, perhaps directing you to a positive outcome or warning you of impending danger, respectively.

This third category is called *clairsentience*, or the ability to know or feel things out of the range of ordinary perception. An unexplained sense of familiarity of having been somewhere, seen something or someone, or heard something before (déjà vu) is representative of this category of *superconsciousness*.

There are several other ways in which you might channel information through physical means. I have a friend who often gets a queasy feeling in her stomach when she is exposed to dishonesty or dark omens. This methodology of perceiving messages through the digestive tract has been unofficially labeled *gut instinct*. Some people acquire knowledge or insight about a person simply by touching a personal item that belonged to them like a key or wristwatch (*psychometry*) or visiting a place where they may have lived or visited often. They are able to pick up data through distinct personal energy vibrations or particles that are still attached to related physical matter. Taste (*clairgustance*) and smell (*clairolfaction* or *clairalience*) are other examples of heightened physical senses used to trigger some kind of message. The scent of an ex-lover's perfume or the taste of grandmother's favorite recipe without any physical stimulus can elicit memories or impressions somehow pertinent to the message at hand.

When you do start to pass on channeled information, regardless of the manner you receive it, it is not unusual that your voice, facial expression, or posture may change. Your delivery may sometimes take on the energy of Spirit channeling through you. With regard to voice, it may have a different accent, tone, or diction; facial appearance as well as corporeal bearing may take on a more confident, nurturing, or emotive affect than what might be your natural inclination. If your delivery is altered by Spirit, it is best not to resist that particular energy and allow it to pass through you as it is transmitted for the message to have a more direct impact on or identification with its intended recipient or audience.

Whichever modality has the highest certainty to transmit the clearest, most appropriate, and most direct signal to a given individual will be the means Spirit chooses to communicate. Spirit knows what format would serve your highest good to receive information and exactly what information is necessary for you to know at any given time. If you are an aficionado of music and lyrics, the most likely method of contact might be clair-audience. Those who are more visually oriented such as photographers, visual artists, film buffs, etc., usually pick up knowledge via clairvoyance. People in the culinary industry or those in the perfume business might be more inclined to get clues via clairgustance and clairolfaction. It is also not unusual to channel wisdom regarding a specific issue in more than one format if Spirit feels that that is the best way for you to comprehend the information. You may be sent a visual dispatch associated with an auditory message. Also the message may be directed to your particular interests. If you are into films, the visual messages may be transmitted as a scene from a motion picture with which you are familiar and from which the meaning of that scene has a direct relationship to the essence of the communiqué. The interpretation of the messages are specifically directed to your frame of mind, your unique interests, and your way of thinking.

Feel free to communicate with Spirit whenever you feel the desire. Some channelers set aside a regular daily, biweekly, or weekly schedule to make contact. Document your exchanges in a journal or on a recording device so that you not only have a means of recalling the messages but also a way to assess your progress at receiving, interpreting, and delivering messages. From time to time, review your records to evaluate how beneficial you found the information to be.

Messages from Dreams

Dreams are another medium for accessing or channeling higher guidance. Through the deep recesses of your psyche, messages are transmitted to inform, support, and guide you. They can be influential in helping you make crucial decisions and solve problems, alerting you about upcoming threats or potential opportunities, supplying you with useful knowledge about career, activities, aspirations, health, hobbies, friends, loved ones or relatives or helping you to view matters with a different, fresher, or more illuminating perspective.

The good news is that everybody dreams. Unfortunately, not all of you remember your dreams, or if you do, you are not always able to consciously extract the intended messages. It is preferable to be cognizant of your dreams to reap the most value; however, even if you are unaware of them, the pertinent subconscious messages are still delivered to your psyche in ways which also benefit you. Their influence might simply be conveyed more potently when you are mindful of your reverie. It would be futile for Spirit to go through all the work of sending you dreams for no apparent reason.

The more you make an effort to focus on dreaming, the more adept you become at recalling and interpreting your dreams. Just like communicating with Spirit, there is a learning curve. And it is not uncommon that when you do start channeling Spirit, your dreams become more lucid, stronger, and more insightful; for when you make it known to the Universe that you are available for interfacing, Spirit will often message you in several contexts, especially your dreams. One valuable approach is to keep a dream journal. Place it by your bedside, and whenever you wake up with a dream in your memory, write it down as promptly and explicitly as you can recall. The sooner you record it, the more likely you are to remember all the particulars. Sometimes the most unusual or trivial details reveal the most relevant information. In other words, try not to edit. Often recording your dream aids you in deciphering the significance of its message.

One of my patients dreamt that he was in deep conversation with a popular movie star who had beautiful long glistening auburn hair. In the dream her hair was a big focus of his attention. In his life he had a friend with the same distinctive hair color. The conversation that he was having with the actress actually pertained to a strained one he was preparing to have with his friend. Somehow the awkwardness, tension, and discomfort were not factors with the actress in his dream, so his subconscious was able to carefully guide him through the essential elements and proper manner to use in communicating with his friend. The starlet was merely a symbol for his friend. Had he not drawn attention to her conspicuous hair color, the essence of the message might have been lost.

Symbols can have a profound significance in dreams, but it is often more important what they represent to the dreamer than their prototypical meaning. Archetypally, red hair usually suggests a demonic character or one with a seductive or guileful nature. In the previous scenario it implied neither of those qualities. Your intuition is usually quite accurate when it comes to analyzing the symbology of your own dreams. The first thought that comes to mind in your interpretation is generally the best and most judicious. If you find yourself spending too much time and effort to assign a particular meaning to your dream, it is most likely the wrong one. If a specific detail or message keeps popping up even after you attempt to dismiss it, you might want to reconsider that one more seriously. Although taking into account archetypal emblems can be helpful in analyzing the meaning of dreams, it is important to trust your own interpretation.

A helpful practice to obtain the most direct assistance from your dreams is to formulate a specific question to Spirit on which you require enlightenment immediately before getting ready to go to sleep. Resolutely tell yourself that you intend to dream concerning that issue and to remember it distinctly when you wake up. This method might also facilitate the interpretation of the dream because it often narrows the focus within the broad range of issues you might be juggling in your life. Knowing in advance what matter the dream might pertain to can be a tremendously helpful shortcut in ascertaining its meaning.

If you are at an impasse in determining the significance of your dream, it might be helpful if you close your eyes, take several deep breaths, relax your body, quiet your mind, calmly ask higher guidance to assist you in interpreting your dream, and wait patiently for some response. The answer quite often comes to you like an epiphany. You might be pleasantly astounded how effective this technique is.

Jeanette had started dating a lawyer. They had only gone out a couple of times, yet she could sense he was more interested in pursuing the physical side of the relationship than she was. At that early stage in their relationship, necking was not enough to satisfy his desire. She liked him socially and intellectually, but she did not feel right about proceeding so fast physically. Her girlfriends were much more uninhibited than she and urged her to loosen up if she wanted to hold on to this man. Insecure and perplexed about her feelings, she decided to ask for guidance via her dreams. That night she dreamt that a girlfriend had phoned her to watch the TV show *Sex and the City*. In her dream, something was malfunctioning with her transmission, and she was unable to watch the show. Instead, she only had reception for the sitcom *Friends*. The dream had confirmed her sentiments: she viewed this man as a friend, but at least at that juncture not as someone with whom she would pursue more romantic endeavors.

Some dreams can be prophetic. Whether they serve to warn you of some impending danger or to impart some useful future knowledge, what you do with that information is up to you. Robert, an optometrist, was fascinated by his dreams. He kept a dream journal and a book on how to interpret his dreams by his bedside. One night he dreamt about a patient whom he had not seen in a long time. In the dream the man was sitting on top of a huge pile of oranges. Robert found the dream very odd, but it was even more uncanny when the guy unexpectedly visited him for a consultation a few days later. Robert knew that the dream was significant but not exactly how and why. He examined the patient more thoroughly than usual because of the circumstances. Curiously he discovered an atypical and obscure finding of *orange* streaks on this man's retina. The patient was developing an extremely rare ocular disease. Had Robert not been forewarned in his dream, he wondered whether he might have missed this vague finding and rare diagnosis altogether.

At another time, Robert was experiencing nightmares. He woke up feeling miserable but could not recall the specific contents of his dreams. What's more, the nightmares lasted a whole week, and the uncomfortable and wretched feelings they elicited felt like doom and persisted during the daytime. He was petrified because he sensed something massively grave, as if his own life were in danger. The day the last nightmare of that ilk ended was September 11, 2001. Robert, a resident New Yorker, was not anywhere near the World Trade Center that day, but his empathic soul was attuned to that nearby impending tragedy.

Meditative Exercise: Connecting with Spirit

The following exercise is a proactive means you can use to familiarize yourself with Spirit. As previously mentioned, since quieting, relaxing, and focusing the mind and thus elevating the vibration of your consciousness are natural byproducts of meditation, this mental discipline often facilitates your connection to an environment with a higher energy vibration compatible with the spirit world. This slightly altered level of consciousness is often described as a trance or channeled state. After much practice with and commitment to this technique, you can become quite adept at entering the channeled state, often within minutes to seconds. It is recommended that you first read through this exercise carefully. Then come back to do it when you have approximately a half hour or more to spare in an undisturbed, quiet, and soothing setting. Prepare to calm both your mind and body. It is preferable that you sit in a comfortable upright position so that your vibration can rise above your crown in order to interface with Spirit's vibration, which must be lowered to match yours.

Start this process by closing your eyes and taking deep slow breaths in through your nose and out through your mouth: both of these acts help relax your system and slow down the frequency of your brainwaves. Then visualize a giant blank white sheet of paper in front of you. On this paper envision posting all your concerns: whether they are about your job, your finances, your romantic partner, your family, your health, politics, even your to-do list, and so on. Now imagine taking this sheet of paper, folding it up, putting it in an envelope, and then placing it in a drawer for approximately a half hour. Next, start to release physical tension by focusing on your body. Systematically move from your toes to your arches, ankles, calves, knees, thighs, pelvis, abdomen, chest, back, shoulders, arms, forearms, hands, fingers, neck, face, and scalp. Take your time. Imagine your muscles as flaccid and relaxed as a jellyfish gently floating underwater while all the stress flows out of each part of your body. Feel your physical form unwind and loosen up.

Next visualize a huge warm golden-orange sun radiating soothing energy above your body. As you inhale, take in some of that calming and nourishing light, and as you exhale, expel as much tense, toxic, heavy, and dark energy as you can. Soon the luminous luster starts to fill and surround your being. You may sense the warmth and glow bathing each and every cell in your body. Periodically rub your palms together gently for brief periods to increase your vibration and facilitate your connection with Spirit. You may feel a tingling sensation in various parts of your body or feel lighter in your frame as if you are floating toward the light. Now breathe deeply and slowly to a count of twenty. When you reach twenty, you should be in a completely relaxed state.

In the next phase of the meditation, imagine yourself traveling upward toward a beautiful and peaceful setting. This place could seem like a favorite beach, lake, river, mountain, garden, or meadow. It may be a location to which you have never been but only dreamt about, or it may resemble a beloved room, home, lodge, castle, boat, church, temple, mosque, ashram, or shrine. Wherever or whatever the place, consider this site your sanctuary now. Nothing bad could ever happen to you there. It is the safest, most serene, most relaxing, and most comfortable haven. You might even imagine some of your favorite soothing and supportive possessions or influences surrounding you in this sanctuary. You might choose some crystals, candles, a preferred comforter, a pillow, some sentimental keepsakes, a talisman, gentle music, or your favorite sounds of nature like the ocean waves.

While you are still in a pleasant state of serenity, imagine an obscure ball of white light off in the distance slowly coming toward you as it increases in size, focus, and luminosity. The light is bright yet soothing, and you perceive it to have pure, loving, healing energy. When it is almost close enough for you to reach out and touch, the light may transform and appear to have some kind of human, animal, alien, mechanical, or other recognizable qualities. You may see, hear, or feel Spirit, or you may even communicate telepathically. Scrutinize Spirit intently. It is full of all the benevolent energy that you had initially perceived in the ball of bright light. Spirit may seem to be male, female, or androgynous, and if you are more prone to a visual impression, may be unadorned or arrayed in ancient garb, more modern attire, or any number of colors and novel coverings. You may feel a sense of recognition, reverence, captivation, or exhilaration. Spirit acknowledges and greets you with deep affection. If you have difficulty perceiving Spirit, kindly ask Spirit to strengthen your link.

Welcome Spirit. Ask for a name. Think of some questions you may want to ask. If you are unsure what is appropriate to inquire, simply request any information that would serve your highest good to know at this juncture in time and space. Do not be disappointed if you do not receive a response straightaway or if you cannot understand the answer. Stay calm. Try to absorb whatever you are feeling, seeing, hearing, or thinking as often the messages come in ways you were not expecting. Some people feel that it is their imagination or a daydream when it is in fact Spirit's manner of connecting with them. Sometimes the messages may come to you later or become clearer with more experience. Be patient and do not put undue pressure on yourself. Bask in as much of the wondrous enlightenment as you are able to perceive being bestowed upon you. Although it varies for each person, when you feel that sufficient time has elapsed for an initial encounter or attempt, thank Spirit for the experience whether you connected or not, and if you feel inclined, extend an open invitation for future meetings. To conclude your meditation, slowly open your eyes, stretch your body, rub your feet on the floor to ground yourself, and start to awaken from your trance state.

First channeling experiences are interesting and varied. The most important fact to note is that there is no right or wrong encounter. Whatever happened during the meditation was exactly what was supposed to. If you did not make a clear or satisfying connection or any contact for that matter, do not despair; this sometimes happens. Just like when you were a young child learning to advance from training wheels to riding a two-wheeled bicycle, some of you might have been successful on the first try and some of you might have taken many more attempts to succeed. Consider trying again. Perhaps you were not relaxed enough. Take a break to contemplate the experience before making another attempt. Remember that if you have the sincere and devoted intention to channel Spirit, it is inevitable that it will happen. Spirit is eager, waiting, and wanting to connect with you. If the encounter was disappointing or not particularly lucid, do not hesitate to ask Spirit to help adjust, strengthen, and improve the connection. Perhaps you may need to put any doubts or fears that you might harbor about this experience aside. If the event was a meaningful and enriching one, congratulations for having formally bonded with a most auspicious relationship. You now have a companion who is ready, able, and devoted to being an excellent source of inspiration, guidance, and wisdom whenever you summon Spirit.

How to Heal with Spirit

Once you have made contact and established a relationship with Spirit, you should never feel alone or lost. Access to help should be simple and convenient. All you need to do is relax your body, quiet your mind, breathe deeply, and ask for guidance. Once a channeling connection is set up, it is never severed and only becomes stronger and more efficient the more you utilize it.

Do not be timid about asking questions, but keep one thing in mind: Spirit responds to matters that would serve your highest good to know. This encompasses a broad range, but if you are uncertain whether your query is appropriate, you can always preface your question with, "Would it serve my highest good to ask or know...?" Some examples of appropriate queries would be: "What do I need to know about my arthritis? Why have I attracted it, and how can I alleviate it?" or "How can I best move forward in my career?" or "What insight can you provide regarding the present difficulties I am having with my partner?" Requesting the winning numbers to this week's lottery jackpot might more than likely not be the best choice of information to seek. The inquirer may certainly feel that the answer to that latter request would serve his or her highest good, but the Universe might have a different opinion. Sometimes a question might seem appropriate, but its reply is denied because the knowledge would not be as beneficial to the individual as actually acquiring it directly from experience. Seeking any insight that might shed light on healing your soul, your mind, your emotions, or your physical body would be a subject of suitable query. That would be a good starting point, although the field of inquisition is more extensive. If the information sought would benefit another person or group or, on a larger scale, humanity, the animal kingdom, or the planet without causing any incidental harm, the focus of the request is most likely quite proper.

Here's a good example of how Spirit was helpful with healing advice. A physician I know was suffering from lower back pain. His symptoms seemed to flare and remit without any obvious discernible cause. He had consulted several back specialists without significant benefit.

Medications, acupuncture, cool compresses, and massage helped to suppress and soothe his symptoms only for brief periods. While talking to him one day, I saw him wince in pain while pressing his lower back with his hand, which led him to tell me about his condition. At that point, I received a vision of the Security Council of the United Nations in session. The room was filled to capacity with delegates. The word *delegate* kept reverberating in my head. It turned out that my colleague was grappling with two problematic issues—being a perfectionist and needing to be in control of everything. Tasks had to be done his way, and there was no wiggle room. If assignments were not carried out specifically as he had mandated, he would simply redo them himself. He also performed several staff chores himself rather than assigning them to employees because he wanted them to be done "correctly." But all this extra workload consumed too much of his time and energy and took its toll on both his mental and physical health. If he had been aware enough to stop and listen to the message that his body was attempting to give him, he might have spared himself much of the time and effort he had spent seeking temporary remedies. Instead, the one true expert on his condition, his soul, had relayed directives to his physical body to transmit a signal to him via his lower back basically saying, "Ease up, man, do not try to take on most of the workload yourself; *delegate* tasks to others." That was the message I shared with him. The pain actually forced him to slow down; he had no choice. The weight of the burden figuratively stressed the muscles in his back as if he were Atlas holding up the world. Finally, because of his intense pain, he was ready to accept and follow the counsel he had been sent, and he learned to *delegate* duties, take the time to instruct others how he wanted things done, and relinquish his expectations of perfection. Not surprisingly, his back no longer pains him. The mind and body and spirit connection can be a mighty effective circuit. Never underestimate it. How wonderful and empowering it is to be able to heal yourself using your very own circuitry!

In this scenario, Spirit transmitted messages utilizing three different modes of channeling: clairvoyance, which dispatched an image of the *delegates* in the Security Council of the United Nations; accompanied by clairaudience, which transmitted the word *delegate*; and finally clairsentience, which delivered the insight elucidating how this man's actions and attitudes were responsible for his back pain.

Destiny and Spiritual Guidance

Many of you seek answers concerning destiny. There is a widely held belief that the future is predetermined. That conception is not completely accurate. You are all given free will to alter your minds, emotions, and actions at any time. The future is based on fluctuating energies and probabilities, not certainties. However, to briefly explain this notion, you must first understand that physical reality is a dynamic system composed of fluctuating particles and waves of energy that exist all around you. Your thoughts, feelings, and actions also belong to that same energy network by which you create your reality in the form of objects, conditions, and experiences. If you alter your thoughts, feelings, and actions, you can change your energy and, hence, your reality. This phenomenon applies to both individuals and groups.

The following two scenarios demonstrate how the energy of thoughts, feelings, and actions can alter your world both on an individual and a mass level.

In regard to how this might affect an individual, suppose an office job that Hank was initially passionate about gradually no longer appealed to him. He still physically performed his job the same way as before but without enthusiasm and pride. Even though he was no longer ardent about his work, he had no intention of quitting and searching for another position. Then one day his boss was promoted and replaced with someone new. The successor did not appreciate Hank or his job performance and fired him. Although Hank was not consciously planning this scenario, the energy of Hank's apathetic attitude toward his job set in motion the changes in his reality that led to his unexpected dismissal.

As an example demonstrating this concept on a group basis, suppose an overwhelming majority of a population has agreed to welcome a large international corporation to a less economically developed area of their city. Both the governor and the mayor have been working hard to attract this company because it would provide many jobs and be a huge boost to the economy. The media has drummed up a lot of excitement concerning this venture. Plans have been set in motion for this to happen, and the public eagerly awaits the corporation's arrival. Yet a small contingent of local neighborhood politicians has begun to voice resistance to this plan because it feels that this huge corporation might negatively impact local long-standing residents not employed by this operation by increasing their cost of living. Slowly but steadily the opposition gains momentum until it has turned the tide of public sentiment against this development, and the corporation eventually backs out of the deal. What once seemed certain to come to fruition is now nonexistent. The overall thoughts, feelings, and actions—hence, the net energy—once highly in favor of creating this venture had shifted quite strongly in the opposite direction. Had not the energy of a small group of committed citizens alerted, influenced, and redirected the widespread consciousness of the aggregate, the future of that city would have been quite different.

In the above scenarios, questioning Spirit about an outcome would have led to wavering responses depending upon the energy of the thoughts, feelings, and actions surrounding each of those situations at the particular time of inquiry. So instead of asking Spirit whether or when an event will occur, it might have been more prudent for the parties involved to seek advice in a broader sense like what would serve their highest good to know and how they could best actualize their goals. The advice for Hank might have been for him to try to rekindle the passion he once had for his job at his present company or search for more inspiring work elsewhere. And if the corporation was strongly seeking to relocate to that city, Spirit might have recommended that it communicate from the start how it planned to make provisions that would benefit the standard of living not only for its potential new employees but also for the longtime inhabitants not in its employ.

A Contract to Heal

To some of you the information that you are about to read in this segment may seem novel and inconceivable. To others it may appear familiar and credible. Whatever your background or prior thoughts, allow your mind to be open. The following concepts do not emanate from any particular spiritual practice or religion, although similar theories can be found throughout various traditions. I am offering these insights because I believe they are resolutely linked to healing. They impart a cosmic and more illuminating perspective of what role healing plays in the broader design of your existence.

Although each of you has been given talents, a soul, emotions, a body, and a mind that allow you to maneuver through a variety of experiences that challenge and encourage you to grow, you are ultimately responsible for choosing your own script in this lifetime. Before you were born, the more senior authorities in the Universe presented your soul with an invitation to visit the earth's physical plane to deal with some of your issues, experience something new, expand your consciousness, and evolve. This is one of the ways in which your soul matures and broadens its repertoire. Before your soul envelops and bonds with the body, it is given choices. These options are akin to an actor choosing a play and character for which to audition. Not every soul is the right fit for a particular role. You might have performed quite successfully in a similar play or part during the last season—your previous lifetime—and repeating the same or a similar performance would not enhance your career unless the previous show was a flop you feel you can amend. In that case, it might be appropriate to take on that role again in order to approach it from a different angle, this time hopefully performing better and receiving more favorable reviews. Once you have done that, you could aim for something different and more challenging in the next gig or lifetime.

So after you have auditioned for the production, obtained the role, signed the contract with the producer—

in this case, the Universe—and rehearsed several ways to perform your part, you are then ready to step into character. At this juncture, just like the actor who has reviewed and studied the entire script, your soul is privy to a complete fund of knowledge of all the relevant events, challenges, good fortunes, achievements, and all the significant people who are to play a part in shaping your life, as well as places such as country of origin, residences, and other noteworthy locales where you are destined to visit.

After the contract is signed, you become so deeply immersed in your script and your persona and so intently focused on the present moment in your character's life that you forget who you were before you assumed that role and the precise course of events in your character's future. That is why there is no prenatal recollection or knowledge as to who or what you were before and how the developments of your life might unfold. The element of free will (how you choose to approach your character in rehearsal and how you act in each performance) is also integrated into the production of your life. But, and this is of utmost importance, it is your mission to remember who you truly are (staying true to your character) and to become who you desire to be (to genuinely evolve and mature into the epitome of your character as the script unfolds).

Of course, this is a loose and simplified metaphorical interpretation of what occurs, but once the final curtain of the last performance comes down, your soul returns from whence it came until it is ready for its next gig. The soul is immortal; you exist eternally, yet simply change physical form and conscious orientation on your many visitations to the earthly dimension. Plays open and close, but there is always time and space before, during, and after productions where essence subsists. Out of sight and out of mind do not connote a void. When a toddler plays the game peekaboo by putting his hands over his eyes and exclaiming, "You cannot see me!" his mind is too naïve to comprehend that just because he cannot perceive others does not mean others cannot see him. Similarly, the fact that you have no recollection or knowledge of your existence before or after physical life does not indicate that that time, place, or state is null and vacant to your soul. It is paramount to learn to open and expand your consciousness just the way the toddler one day will.

You, via your soul, come into physical form to evolve, heal deep-rooted issues, become more enlightened, broaden your awareness, experience the gamut of worldly existence, create fresh ideas and substance, remember who you are, and pursue becoming who you want to be. You will never truly arrive at your ultimate journey's end or become the vision of your soul's apotheosis, for you are continuously attempting to reach new heights. It is like exploring outer space: once you have reached one destination, there will always be another more distant and challenging one to target and explore. You persist in making efforts to return in order to surpass your previous goals. Just as there are other planets and galaxies to seek out and investigate, there are other realities, dimensions, and incarnations in which to travel, better yourself, and experience being beyond the one you know in this lifetime.

At the soul level, you strive for adventure, expansion, and challenge. When you are growing and experiencing life in a wonderful way, you feel healthy and strong. When you are constricted, stuck, or faltering, your soul attempts to redirect you by sending you messages in the form of symptoms, signs, dreams, or edifying circumstances. You are given several opportunities to make changes and forge ahead by means that enrich and nurture the soul. The Universe truly hopes that you can and will succeed. If you do not, there is no shame or dishonor; the Universe does not judge, for it knows that you are like a child attempting to find the light through the darkness. It is similar to the student who is left back a grade because of failure to achieve a certain level of competency and command of subject matter: a being might be requested to return to an equivalent physical existence to grasp certain issues and experiences necessary for its evolution at that juncture before moving on to the next level. In the repeat performance, the associated characters and events might be different, but the fundamental issues are the same. And like the protagonist, some of the cohort souls may be returning for similar reasons.

Whether you are returning with former friends, enemies, lovers, siblings, or parents, these beings can take on different roles in each of your lifetimes. In other words, someone who was your father in one lifetime may take on the part of your brother in another. Souls are also androgynous. Your sister two lifetimes ago may be your husband or brother in another. There is a proclivity to return with a core constellation of familiar souls. Not all of them will appear in each lifetime, but over many lifetimes there is a pattern of a principal group of former kindred spirits reuniting just as some actors, directors, choreographers, costume designers, sound technicians, and producers seem to reconnect and collaborate on several different projects. You long to be with familiar souls and spur each other on in development. On some level, you may recognize these fellow returning souls in a déjà vu phenomenon; you may feel a certain level of comfort with them or perhaps even experience an uneasiness with them that you may wish to have the chance to resolve.

Your journey of healing, therefore, does not just take place during this lifetime. The soul is immortal, and healing transcends many lifetimes. Each of your incarnations is designed to give you more opportunities to heal and grow. Features of your past lives may help you understand why you are confronting particular issues in your present existence, yet what is of paramount importance is the need to experience, evolve, and heal in the here and now. So once you have been dealt your cards in your present lifetime, it is up to you to forge the best outcome. And be aware that everyone comes to life from different playing fields and with unique agendas. To make comparisons and draw conclusions for your own life based upon the substance of anyone else's is futile. You are a single entity beginning at your own distinct starting point, moving at your own special pace, being true to your own unique interpretation of life, and acting on your own free will.

One of the most important prerequisites to establishing a spiritual connection is to have an open mind, which leads to the next level on which you can heal.

⟋ 4 ⟍

Healing on a Mental Level

The Workings of the Mind

You literally are what you think. What you think, you communicate; what you communicate, you do; what you do, you experience; what you experience, you become; what you become, you are; and what you are, you think. The mind spins a loop that sets the stage for you to press on. It is all up to you as to who you want to be, what you want to create, where you want to go, how you want to proceed, and why you should bother.

What you ponder and believe creates your reality. On one level it seems so simplistic and natural, yet on another it sounds quite hypothetical and unfathomable. The mind is a very powerful entity. Never underestimate it: it is responsible for conceiving and generating all that appears in your world, good and bad. It is best to be most careful how and what you contemplate, because you may have to live with its consequences. It is best to develop a close and congenial relationship with the mind; if you treat it with kindness, respect, and firmness, understand and discern its functions, appreciate its presence, and employ it to serve your highest good, it will prove to be a most invaluable and rewarding partner.

Of the four domains in which you heal, the mind is the one requiring the most vigorous molding. From the start, the physical body was and still is sending you constructive signs; the soul, whether you are aware of it or not, is always directing you toward the light; and your emotions have consistently allowed you to know and connect with your truth. Yet when you first encountered the mind, it was in its novice stages—relatively unrefined compared to the other three healing dimensions. With proper instruction and coaching, the mind can be a most indispensable ally, helping you communicate and collaborate more adroitly and effectually with the other three dimensions of your being. Just because your mental faculty first approached you untamed does not diminish its value or significance as an essential component of who you are.

In order to better understand this complex mental element, it is best to view it in relation to the other essential components of your being. When doing this, there are usually two schools of thought: the consolidators and the dividers, otherwise known as the lumpers and the splitters. The former have a tendency to bunch entities and ideas together in order to simplify their meaning and purpose. For the latter the opposite is true: teasing apart the affiliated yet distinct associations from an entity in order to allow its uniqueness and pith to stand alone. Recognizing more defined and discrete identities can sometimes offer a clearer understanding of perplexing subjects. The prevailing holistic dogma that subdivides the origins of the health and disease continuum into the trilogy of "mind, body, and spirit" either combined or overlooked a major category—emotions. When referring to the mind, body, and spirit, I feel that it is helpful to distinguish the cognitive, physical, and spiritual components from the more visceral one with regard to healing. Although the mental and affective segments are similar, they clearly have distinct and separate roles. I use the terms *mental* when referring to the cognitive faculties like reason and intellect, *emotional* when pertaining to more passionate sensibilities like love and fear, *physical* when dealing with concrete and tangible aspects like organs and tissues, and *spiritual* when alluding to transcendental elements like the soul and the afterlife. Subsequent chapters will deal with healing on the emotional and physical levels.

The mind is where you formulate your beliefs. It determines how you view the world. All the unique volitional qualities that contribute to who you are course through the mind. Whether it is the career you have selected, the activities you choose to participate in, the traits you exhibit, the people you associate with, or the style you exude, the common thread stitching together who you are is your mind. Like the body, the mind is always in a state of flux. As you mature and evolve, your opinions are likely to change. What was once firmly embedded in your consciousness may shift as you experience disillusioning outcomes or are exposed to fresh, appealing, and innovative ideas. Your belief system is constantly remodeling itself as old and new convictions are repeatedly scrutinized. If you should decide that part of you is no longer compatible with your ideas of who you want to be, you must first return to the mind to make the necessary adjustments. There is no right or wrong—only what fits best or is incongruous at a particular moment with regard to who you are or want to be. For example, Jane was once an unmitigated conservative and Republican, but developed more liberal and Democratic Party views after she witnessed the discomfiting harsh realities of a war fueled by a Republican administration.

The mind is invisible. It is not matter, yet it can affect matter. It is energy. It produces thought, and thought is energy. It resides in every cell of your body. It seems as though the mind is solely in the brain because that is where there is the densest concentration of cells and the highest consumption of energy, but it is just the busiest processing center. Each cell of your body has its own consciousness. It is in your body's cells that the energy which is your thought is translated and converted into physical effects.

The energy of the mind is mighty potent. Almost like magic, what it dwells on, you tend to attract. Energy attracts energy of an equivalent nature. It is important to be prudent about all potential conceptualizations and images you attach to your charged mental matrix. Make a concerted effort to release from the mind all that is undesirable and to hold on to all that you seek. The more time, attention, and effort spent deliberating on specific thoughts and perceptions—good or bad—the greater the power they accrue, and the greater the probability you will attract them into your reality. You have the capability to improve your mind by the way you develop and groom it. When the quality of your thoughts rises to a high level, your consciousness becomes more evolved and its vibration increases. Therefore, when you elevate the vibration of your mind by upgrading your thoughts, you are also capable of attracting other energies of an equivalent higher vibration which can be demonstrated as improved opportunities, abilities, assets, sentiments, and health.

This was clearly demonstrated to me in my own life. In the latter part of 2013, I was seeking to expand my channeling clientele beyond select medical patients and friends. A person I had recently met introduced me to a hospital chaplain she thought would be amenable to allowing me to volunteer my channeling services to his hospitalized clients. When I first met with this chaplain at his rectory, he seemed to be totally oblivious and unreceptive to the concept of channeling until I took the time to explain its principles, means, and objectives. Afterward he politely offered to confer with his senior colleagues to see if something could possibly be arranged and said he would get back to me with a response within two weeks. When the two-week deadline had passed and I did not hear from him, I left a message for him to contact me. A week later I left a second message. Not only was I disappointed and dejected that he did not follow up, but also that my dreams surrounding this hopeful prospect were quashed. It took about another week for me to put my discontented feelings concerning this missed opportunity aside and press on, and then something extraordinary happened. Out of the blue an esteemed mentor and friend contacted me to inform me that she had decided to retire from her channeling practice of thirty years and wondered if I would be interested in taking on her clients. My wishes to broaden my channeling pursuits that I had been transmitting to the Universe must have been highly charged, for they were undoubtedly granted in ways far better than I could have imagined.

There are basically three ways in which the mind functions regarding creating reality. In the most reliable and beneficially precise scenario, you must be resolute and proactive in directing the mind to focus on exactly who you want to be, what you want to do, or what you want to contrive. In a second option, your thoughts are active, but they are constantly fluctuating, thereby delaying or inhibiting any reality from launching from them. And in the third case, your thoughts are passive and undecided, and you indirectly allow the collective consciousness to dictate what the mind attracts.

With regard to the first way, when you take an active role in cognition, you tend to procure what you contemplate as long as you keep your mind fixed and intent on your goals. The time element is variable and tricky, though, because much depends not only on how well you are able to concentrate but also on the nature of your goals. Further on in this chapter I plan to discuss meditation, a process which can help train your mind to be still and focused, and the art of manifestation, a more detailed approach for mindfully creating your own reality. The person who consistently ponders and communicates bonhomie seems more often than not to attract pleasurable situations, and the one who is routinely thinking or talking about doom and gloom is more likely to create unpropitious circumstances.

A variant of this first mental manifesting method encompassing a multitude of minds is called collective thinking, akin to collaborative prayer. It is a process whereby many minds are working together with similar thoughts and goals. The combination of the duration and energy expended multiplied by the number of active minds focusing on a central idea creates a highly effective and powerful way to transform cogitation into reality. Typical examples of this phenomenon resulted in the legalization of women's right to vote in the United States in 1920 and the dismantling of the Iron Curtain in the late 1980s and early 1990s. Granted, depending on the nature of the objective, the time span for enough energy to accumulate to manifest it can be considerable as is apparent in the two aforementioned examples.

The second type of scenario of mental actualization addresses situations where ideas are constantly being altered. In such instances mixed messages are being transmitted into your energy field until it becomes a confusing and unaccommodating environment for any notions to manifest. It is akin to changing your prerequisites with regard to the type of home you are looking to purchase. First you decide on a freestanding house far from the city with five bedrooms and a large yard. Later you realize that the commute and upkeep on that choice are not preferable, so you alter your terms to a four-bedroom town house closer to the city with a shorter commute. For a more convenient lifestyle, next you consider a three-bedroom apartment within the city center. Needless to say, your real estate agent is having a difficult time finding you prospects. You might even come to the conclusion after all the effort and indecision to postpone your plans to move until you feel more confident in your objectives. Think how confusing and difficult it is for your mind to help manifest what you want when you are not even sure what that is. In this second scenario, ideas seem to take longer spans of time, if ever, to manifest.

The third possibility occurs when your mind is neither decided nor deliberating options but rather stays empty and, hence, attaches to the collective consciousness—the combined energy or thoughts of an attendant group or culture. An example of this would be Abe consenting to join the family business after graduating from college based on his family's opinion that it would be a sound decision. At that juncture he was not particularly passionate about or considering any specific career, but since his father, mother, uncle, and grandfather all agreed, Abe was inducted into the family business. The truth is that he never really liked that career choice, but since his mind was not committed to any other option he aligned with the familial or collective consciousness by default. Years later he did eventually become enthused about a different vocation. At that juncture, he actively focused his mind on and pursued his ambition, and thereafter bowed out of his ancestral trade.

There is a whole gamut of functions and byproducts that make up the mind: ideas, creativity, imagination, memories, reflections, confusion, negativity, narrowness, delusions, inventions, knowing, learning, logic, and brilliance to name a few and acquaint you with just how grand this entity is. It is an amazing and complex system where so much is happening beneath the surface. At times it functions and delivers like a well-maintained machine, and at other times, the results do not seem to provide what is desired. But as with any instrument or system, there are methods and practices that aid as well as ones that hinder it in working to your advantage. Getting to know the mind is no easy feat. It is a challenging process, but with some practical information, useful techniques, and a broader perspective, you can truly gain some mindful mastery to improve and ease your relationship with it.

Your relationship with the mind can be similar to one you may have with a cherished pet like a dog, who can be loyal, loving, and smart, as well as disruptive, exhausting, and stubborn. It is wise to get to know it and build a relationship with it so that it can serve you in amazing ways. Be sure to inform it who is in charge. Be clear as to what you expect from it. Speak your mind as well as speak to your mind. Observe how it operates.

Instruct it to help you through use of beneficial practices—affirmations, meditation, appropriate semantics, the art of manifesting your reality—described later in this chapter. Guide it, respect it, and nurture it. Express your gratitude when it responds well to your directives. Inform it and redirect it when it acts in ways not of your liking. Rest it when it is tired. Send it calming energy and soothing words and thoughts when it is irritable. Advise and teach it to desist or slow down when it is overactive and overwhelming and draining your energy. And most important, be thankful to have it as your companion.

The mind is mighty. The question is who is in control, you or it? Should the horse or the carriage driver be in charge? Should the bride and groom or the wedding planner be making final decisions? If you know what you want and where you want to go and feel competent, take the helm, but work respectfully together as you would with any valued member of a team. The more in control you are of the whole process when dealing with your mental mogul, the more your journey will be a smoother, calmer, and more enjoyable experience. Take the extra time to think, plan, focus, and decide who you are and what you want, so that the mind can follow your directives and does not need to be a mind on its own.

Affirmations

One way to work with the mind to your advantage is to develop a positive and favorable set of beliefs and statements called affirmations. More than just an unequivocal and beneficial declaration, an affirmation is an empowering claim and forthright assertion. These phrases guide your psyche in the direction you wish to feel, be, and act. If channeled properly, affirmations have the capability to create a shift in your aura or the energy that surrounds you to help create the changes in your life that you seek.

The first matter of business is to devise or find an encouraging statement that fulfills a significant elemental need in your life. One important rule is that there be no expression of limitation, negative connotation, or with rare exceptions, any negating words as part of the phrase. For example, if you often feel timid and desire to change that state of mind, you can simply assert, "I am a confident being, and I am becoming more bold and self-assured each day." You may conceive one or more affirmations, but try not to overload your mind with more than two or three at any one period of time. Choose subjects which are most relevant and pressing. Once they have served their purpose, you can create new ones and work on other issues.

Keep your affirmations clear, simple, and to the point. Run-on sentences and elaborate, complex words or phrases tend to detract from the crux of the message. It is much like when you are attending a lecture and too much information is disseminated in a short span of time; it becomes too burdensome for your mind to assimilate and retain all the significant details.

Your gut feeling must be comfortable and confident about the affirmation. Does it seem uplifting, supportive, sound, and likely to promote growth? If the overall message or the words do not feel right, change them.

Stick to the present tense. Keeping the mind focused on the here and now is the most powerful means to impress messages on it. All that you ever experience is the present moment; it is the most potent and direct for you, because the past has occurred and the future is not yet here. The present holds a fresh clean slate from which to be. Right now you have the potential and power to create anything you desire. Assume that and behave as if your declaration is already true, for once your mind is convinced of this, your affirmation is becoming a reality.

But if the Universe is aware that your consciousness harbors doubt and hesitation, you have sent a message that you are not completely ready to claim your proposal, because it was just that, not a pronouncement. This may reflect some inner conflict, fear, or apprehension about change or moving forward in your life. These feelings are natural. Try not to be upset with yourself. Conceivably you might have chosen to tackle more than you were prepared for at that juncture and might need to take smaller steps. Only you can decide how you want to proceed. But because you have even considered working with affirmations, you have already made some sort of statement that you want to evolve, advance, and better yourself—and that is a great first step. I encourage you to take some extra time to reflect and perhaps modify your statement, regroup, and reaffirm.

Sharon, a young woman in her late twenties, was struggling with an eating disorder. Sharon's father, a physician who placed a great deal of emphasis on health, diet, and fitness, doted on his only daughter and would often make comments regarding her food choices, exercise regimen, and the weight and tone of her body. Dealing with low self-esteem and boyfriend issues, Sharon channeled all her energy and attention into eradicating all fat and junk food from her diet and exercising regularly to create the perfect body. That was one area of her life in which she felt that she was able to excel and be in control. What started out with good intentions turned extreme. Her weight management and exercise routine became a predominant focus of her existence. She lost the ability to view her body realistically. Her physique eventually appeared emaciated, and she developed anemia, amenorrhea, hair loss, and fatigue. At that point she agreed to seek medical assistance and psychotherapy. Around the same time, a close and loving friend provided her with a card printed with the affirmation, "I love and appreciate my body just the way it is," and told her to refer to it as often as she could. Because of her deep respect and admiration for her friend, she kept the card and looked at it from time to time but did not hold much belief in its potential to do her any good. Many months, added pounds, and therapy sessions later when she was at the gym preparing to exercise and listen to music on the treadmill, she shuffled through the contents of her bag to locate her headphones to no avail. She did however come upon the affirmation card her friend had given her. While running on the treadmill and facing a full-length mirror mounted on the wall in front of her, she kept repeating the affirmation in her head. During that workout something suddenly clicked and shifted for Sharon in an extraordinary moment of insight. Twenty pounds above her nadir while staring at her body in the mirror, she realized how much she loved her legs and hips and buttocks just the way they were. She is now able to see the full beauty of her body and nurture and cherish it in a healthy way.

The next step is to make your affirmations a part of your day. You can write them in your journal, recite or sing them out loud or silently in your head, or post them in conspicuous places. One helpful practice is to print your affirmations clearly on several index cards. Then place them in a number of prominent locations: on your night table next to your alarm clock so you can see them before you retire and as soon as you awaken, on your refrigerator door, on your bathroom mirror, in your reading material as a bookmark, on your desk, in your billfold, on your bulletin board, or wherever you pass frequently. The more you notice them, the more you read them, and the more you impress their messages upon your mind, the more likely they are to ultimately become a reality. Repetition is an important element in their actualization.

You should heed your affirmations until you feel that you have achieved a sufficient and satisfying level of progress in your objectives. It does not matter whether it takes one month, one year, or even longer to occur as long as it does. Headway may be incremental and sometimes difficult to discern. Everyone heals in their own time and on their own personal schedule. There is no such thing as a competition or a deadline when it applies to healing. None of you are identical when it pertains to your issues, your backgrounds, or your psychological constitutions, so why should you expect to heal exactly the same way?

Working with affirmations can do wonders. It is important to be open to new approaches and to have a positive outlook that all things are possible. Simply place your concentration on how you desire to be and be prepared to experience that. Do not be surprised at how amazing and wonderful it is to have the power to heal by changing your perspective.

Affirmations resonate to many different needs and problems. They can be very broad or quite specific. What makes them so valuable and effective is that no matter what the circumstance, they possess a positive way to deal with numerous imaginable issues. The following is a list of several valuable affirmations that cover prevalent and significant themes:

- I am continuously healing and attracting health.

- I now have enough time, energy, money, wisdom, and health to accomplish all my goals.

- I am now attracting loving, fulfilling, happy, healthy, and trusting relationships in my life.

- The Universe is full of abundance, and I am welcome and grateful to share in it.

- I am thankful to have an incredible job where I perform excellent work for which I receive wonderful pay.

- When I encounter a problem fearlessly, there is *no* problem to face. (This is a rare exception of using a negating word as part of the phrase.)

Feel free to use any of these affirmations or conceive some that have more specific relevance to you.

The Energy of Words to Heal

Never underestimate the power of words to heal. Language is a potent force in your lives. What you say and write has a lot to do with what you attract and create. Words can uplift and empower you as well as weaken and defeat you. A large part of the energy that you emit is in the form of communication.

Think carefully and wisely before you speak and choose your words because you just may have to live with their consequences. There are countless times I have heard people use negative, discouraging, and self-deprecating statements in the heat of some emotional turmoil like "I wish I were dead," or "I cannot do anything right," or

"Nobody will ever love me," or "I am pathetic and hope-less!" Those comments are enough to bring anyone down and often represent a warped or exaggerated version of what is fleetingly believed to be the truth. What's more, they bolster a defeatist mentality that makes the process of healing that much more difficult. It is alright to be in touch with your dispirited feelings, but it is also important to be clearly aware and voice that what you are express-ing in a brief moment is often provisional.

After you have finished experiencing your disheart-ened sentiments, try to think of more hopeful, inspir-ing, and encouraging words to express to raise you out of the doldrums. Words can do that. They possess pow-erful energy that has great potential to shift your mood and steer you in an entirely different direction. Look at the statement, "I feel upset that I did not do well on the exam, but next time I plan to study harder and do bet-ter." In the former part of the declaration, both a genu-ine emotion and a fact are expressed. The latter portion introduced by the conjunction *but* alters the drift of the phrase. Now there is a positive intention and a deter-mined expectation of a favored outcome. Your choice of words plays a key role in what influence and power you possess to change your attitude and script your future.

The way that words are expressed, spoken, written, or chanted generates distinct energy, which consequently has great potential to demonstrate and create what they convey. If you catch yourself communicating something that does not feel right, simply retract it and make the necessary corrections. You may indicate that you erred in saying a certain phrase or expressing a particular thought; what you now mean to articulate is something different. You might make the same blunder more than once, and with each rectification, you move closer and closer to the place in your mind you aspire to until you find yourself seamlessly proclaiming exactly what that is. Everyone errs and has the right to change their minds and words. Be kind and gentle to yourself. In a scene out of a conversation from my own life, I inadvertently stated, "*If* my book is published, I plan to. . ." Fortunately the friend I was talking to picked up on my semantic slip as I revised my statement to begin the phrase, "*When* my book is published." The fact that you are now reading this book is proof enough that the subtleness of the words you choose has a powerful impact in actualizing your aspirations.

Angela is a magazine beauty and fashion editor in her early thirties who was exceedingly concerned with her moles. With dark hair, dark eyes, an olive complexion, a modest amount of sun damage for her age, and no family history of skin problems, she did not appear to be at high risk for developing skin cancer. She would make appointments more often than the norm to have her skin examined. "I am worried that I might have skin cancer," she would utter as she pointed to the several moles that concerned her. Sure enough on one of her frequent visits, she did indeed have a melanoma on her back.

It could be deduced that either she was more intuitively in tune with the state of her physical body or her thoughts and words created her disease. Angela did possess prescient faculties, but they pertained more to her areas of expertise than health. She was renowned in her industry for successfully forecasting beauty and fashion trends. Her musings about her physical health veered more toward a preoccupation than a prophecy. Diseases are caused by minds *ill at ease*. Disharmony of a corporeal nature might indicate some kind of mental malaise.

Words and thoughts carry potent energy. People who talk and ruminate about ailments invariably attract them. What she was obsessing about she did indeed acquire. Her scenario reminds me of an old joke—with no intention to make light of Angela's condition—about the hypochondriac whose tombstone was inscribed with the epitaph, "See, I knew I had something serious! Now do you believe me?" The melanoma was surgically removed, and she has been cancer-free for about two decades. Having been informed of the semantic overtones of her speech, she now thinks more judiciously and chooses her words more prudently.

A powerfully wise and edifying statement that deals with the nature of semantics and metaphysical principles deserves mention:

> The words you cast others have a way of
> returning to their origin like a boomerang;
> curse others and you are sure to be
> defeated by your own arrows, but
> comment on their attributes and take notice how
> those graces may well return to you.

You need only look at examples within your own community to recognize the validity of this statement. In regard to those who speak of others with derogatory intent, it is not necessary to identify anyone specifically, but you may recall one or more individuals fitting the following descriptions: the lawmaker indicted for the corruption against which he or she once vociferously fought, the pontificating moralist caught performing an immoral act, and the politician behaving in the same way he or she accused their opponent of acting. Examples of those who speak favorably of others also abound: the spouse who remarks on the virtues of his or her beloved is blessed and showered with their love, and the teacher who uplifts and praises his or her students for their progress and achievements is revered and celebrated.

The Art of Manifestation

By way of thoughtful declarations, coveted conceptualizations, directed efforts, and heartfelt appreciation, manifestations represent what you desire to create in your life. They also represent the ways you attain and complete your plans, goals, and even life purpose. A crucial factor of why you are alive in physical form is to create—either in substance or experience—and what better way to assist you in doing so than by understanding the art of manifestation!

Manifestations and affirmations are not the same, yet they do share subtle features in common. Manifestations are concerned with obtaining something of a more specified, concrete, or circumstantial nature, while affirmations tend to focus on more abstract qualities like cognitive or emotional states. Someone may affirm, "I am now attracting sincere, healthy, and loving relationships in my life," and another individual may record in his journal that he specifically wants to meet people who work in the fields of science and technology, live in Chicago, and are wealthy, college-educated, and athletic. As illustrated in the latter manifestation, the target is more specific about the external attributes regarding what is wanted. In the affirmation, the person's main objective is to attract and surround himself with people whose energies are aligned with his own internal essence. He desires to cherish and be appreciated by others with similar values and philosophies of life, not necessarily particular hobbies, interests, or backgrounds. They both deal with relationships, but manifestations, on a more extrinsic level, and affirmations, on a more inherent, essential, and internal dimension.

To initiate this process, set a specific intention on a substance or a happening which you desire. Whatever you contemplate materializing in your life is the critical element. You may envision a specific type of job, car, apartment, event, or have special and unique requirements when seeking a friend, lover, or pet. Imagine them in the clearest and most precise way possible. Visualize them as if you were creating them in your dreams. Think of the color, texture, shape, size, smell, feel, and taste of the possessions or situations you so desire. Do not edit yourself. Even if you do not have a definite idea as to how your goals and desires might come into being, keep conceptualizing your prime scenario. What you envision will help create the necessary circumstances for your plan to manifest. If you desire a 1965 red Mustang convertible with standard transmission, black leather bucket seats, and white racing stripes on the sides of the chassis, then that is what you must keep in your mind.

It is helpful to record and verbalize your manifestations. This empowers and reinforces them to materialize by utilizing another way to keep their energy vibrant. Devise your own way of creatively expressing your thoughts that is clear and unique to you. No strict rules apply. You may choose to record them in a journal, notebook, or computer. Draw a picture, paste cutouts from a magazine onto a vision board, photograph or videotape them or a likeness thereof, compose a song exhilarating them, or capture their essence in a poem. Review and voice your records often in order to keep their energy fresh and active: the more times your mind registers them, the more energy they accrue and the more effectively they can actualize.

You must not attach to the way your goals may come into being. Some appear in totally unexpected ways, while others seem to arrive more predictably. Much depends on the nature of and the dedication exhibited toward what you want.

Another important element in securing your manifestation is to take action. Besides thinking and recording, when the necessary preconditions appear, you must make an effort to act on them to procure what you want. If you are looking for a humorous romantic partner and a friend invites you to be a guest in his comedy class, do not decline the invitation—by all means go. Do not assume that a jocular mate is magically going to knock at your front door and announce, "You summoned me, now here I am!"

And just as you would expedite affirmations, it is important to harbor a sense of faith. You must truly believe that the forces that create what you are manifesting are set in motion in the present moment; trust and release all doubt. And in addition to knowing that the event or object of your desire is literally on its way toward you, allow the feeling of gratitude to envelop you, which further confirms to the Universe that your mind is clear and confident concerning what you are about to receive.

The following true story demonstrates the power of one Texan family's ability to manifest exactly what they were wishing for. A nine-month-old boy named Justin lost his father to the war in Iraq in 2003. Although he was reared by a loving mother, there was always a part of him that felt a deep void and need to connect with anything that would make him feel closer to his deceased father. Sometime shortly before his fifteenth birthday he told his mother that he wanted a car, but not just any car: he wanted the one his father used to drive. Unfortunately, his mother had sold the father's 1999 Toyota Celica convertible soon after the dad passed. She was no longer aware of its whereabouts. Knowing that somehow finding the father's old car and buying it back would bring Justin inexplicable joy, she decided to post a message online describing the situation, even posting the old VIN of the car, and asking for help in her quest. Miraculously a good Samaritan named Kyle, who resided as far away as Utah and happened to run a charitable organization, read the post and located the car. With the help of donations that he raised, Kyle was able to purchase the car and enlist a team of volunteer mechanics to restore it. This angel of a man personally drove the car from Utah to Texas to surprise Justin on his fifteenth birthday. Justin was overcome with such deep heartfelt and grateful emotions that he was literally at a loss for words. For most people a car is only a material object, but for Justin this car represented so much more—a sentimental link to his father whom he hardly knew but always dreamed of somehow or someday feeling closer to by holding on to one of his most significant and cherished possessions.

Meditation and Healing

Meditation is an acquired introspective discipline that trains the mind to be calm, aware, focused, and refreshed. The benefits extend well beyond the meditative state. Think of it as a routine mental exercise to keep the mind healthy, vital, and fit. It can take many forms. Classically it is practiced in a serene and still environment, but it can also be carried out while focusing on an activity like a walk in the park, listening to music, or gardening. The objective is to allow your mind to concentrate on a specific object, task, issue, or goal such as the flame of a candle, a creative project, a health matter, or a job search, while gently and decidedly emptying it of interfering thoughts, worries, and internal chatter. There are no absolute rules regarding time span or frequency—choose whatever arrangement feels right to you. In that regard, I find wry irony in a quote I've read from Sukhraj S. Dhillon: "You should sit in meditation for twenty minutes every day unless you are too busy; then you should sit for an hour." Like any new application, some of you will take to it more readily and effortlessly than others, but with persistence and practice, each of you is assured to benefit in some way.

Paying attention to your breathing is important no matter what form of meditation you do. Since the mind and the respiratory system work in unison, as your breathing begins to lengthen, your brainwaves begin to slow down. This effect tends to transport you to deeper and more relaxed states of consciousness. Your respirations can also serve as a focal point for your attention, which allows you to clear your mind and release your intrusive thoughts while connecting you to the present moment and guiding your mind back when it may wander away. Following your breath in and out of your body relaxes the mind as well as the body in a way that you can calmly observe and respond to the world around you rather than mindlessly reacting to stimuli. What's more, mindful breathing is a beneficial practice you can do wherever you are and whatever else you are engaged in even when you are not meditating.

Irrespective of the amount of time you are willing or able to devote to meditation, with continued effort and practice there is a resultant overall more serene quality to the mind. You become more conscious of your mind and are able to discover and appreciate the quiet and stillness within. The mind gradually becomes less attached to things that it cannot control like stresses, intrusive thoughts, and stimuli from the external world and develops less affinity to the ego. It becomes less bothered by petty annoyances and is more concerned with what is truly important. In the higher states of consciousness achieved via meditation, your mind becomes more attuned to thoughts related to higher frequencies like confidence and less attuned to those of denser energies like cynicism.

Meditation helps train the mind to be in the here and now or in a state of mindfulness. When the mind meanders to thoughts of the past and the future, it has more opportunity to associate with fretfulness, brooding, and failure. And what's more, when it is more attuned to the present, it is much more conscious of what is going on in its environment—situations and perceptions it might have previously ignored. For some of you it may seem as if you are using a part of your mind you had neglected. It is like your consciousness is now attaching to a floodlight that shines on your environment. Once that light has been established, the mind is able to concentrate on what is directly in front of it more easily, more thoroughly, and more effectively. Remember that time in middle school English class when the teacher suddenly called on you to answer a question about the interpretation of one of Shakespeare's sonnets she had just recited and you were clueless. You were conscious, but your mind was otherwise absorbed daydreaming about what you considered to be more pertinent, more pleasurable, or more interesting, like the new bicycle you were hoping to get for your birthday. Your ears actually heard the poem; however, the words and their meaning did not register in your consciousness. Your purpose for being in that class-room had been diverted. Meditation can help train your mind to concentrate more directly on the present environment with less likelihood of digression to unintended stimuli or thoughts of either the past or the future.

One favorable potential consequence of routine meditation practice is an awareness of a separateness between you and your mind. You gradually come to the realization that you are the true master over your opinions and urges. You are not your thoughts; your mind is an instrument for you to use, not the other way around. In that regard, you have the ability to choose your musings, ideas, and opinions as well as to direct your mind's behavior. For instance, if what you initially liked about a candidate no longer seems right, return to the mind to change its viewpoint. If you do not want your mind to attach to worrisome thoughts, simply redirect it to focus on what you do want. And if it does err, as can be expected at the inception of any new training period, kindly *remind* your mind until its conduct complies instinctively. Just like disciplining a dog to heel during walks, your mental realm can also be conditioned to behave.

When the mind is clear of noise and needless meandering thoughts, it has more serenity, concentration, awareness, and energy to carry out or express a variety of important functions such as learning, creativity, intuition, logic, analysis, and invention, to name a few. Meditation therefore creates a more favorable and comfortable environment whereby the mind is overall better able to serve you and work as a more focused, refreshed, and efficient unit.

Meditation can bring about an aura of serenity, clarity, stability, and revitalization that pervades your entire system. What helps the mind can also positively affect those other dimensions of your being to which it is intimately bound. A whole host of physical, emotional, and spiritual health benefits have been demonstrated as a result of the practice of meditation such as lowering blood pressure, decreasing sensitivity to pain, improving insomnia, increasing willpower to avoid addictions such as alcohol and food binging, increasing feelings of kindness, compassion, and self-esteem, lowering feelings of depression and anxiety, improving stress-related conditions such as inflammatory bowel disease and post-traumatic stress disorder, and enhancing intuition. A healthy body, a sound mind, an available spirit, and wholehearted emotions are some of the magnificent byproducts of a meditative discipline.

Meditative Exercise: Healing

The following exercise is designed to assist you in becoming more comfortable with the practice of meditation. The theme of this particular meditation deals with healing. Before you begin this meditation, set an intention of something that or someone who could benefit from healing. It may be directed toward yourself, a friend, family member, figurehead, pet, garden, or area of the world in need of healing like a war-torn country or an island ravaged by a hurricane. All choices are perfectly acceptable. Meditation is also like a prayer that can be dispatched to all the initiator envisions. Merely focus your intention on the object or representation of whom or what you wish to heal.

Put aside approximately twenty minutes and select a quiet and tranquil location conducive to relaxation. Set any potentially disruptive electronic devices such as computers, phones, or answering machines off or on mute so that you will not be disturbed, and kindly inform any of your housemates to please refrain from making noise and interrupting you until you have completed your task. In the beginning, having the proper environment is a key factor, but with practice you may advance to a point where you are even able to do this routine in a more active setting. Hydrating your body with water before commencing is recommended since often the mouth and nasal mucosa become dry with prolonged deep respirations. Most important, be patient with yourself. If you are having trouble relaxing or clearing your mind, it is alright and quite natural at first. Try not to get upset or frustrated. You may gently follow your distracting thoughts until they exit your consciousness and then resume, or if it is just too trying, simply return to meditate another time when your mood feels more agreeable to the exercise. But remember that with practice you can improve your skills, so the more you meditate, the more adept you can become at it. I do not feel that there are any absolute rules to meditation. What works for some practitioners may not work for others. The following are some helpful hints and useful suggestions to assist you in your meditation:

1. Try to keep your back straight to enhance the flow of energy through your body. You may sit in a chair, on a bed, or on the floor. Although lying on your back or stomach may work for some people, it is

not always ideal for everyone as certain individuals become so relaxed in those positions that they tend to fall asleep. If your positioning allows, place your hands on your thighs with your palms facing up. Form two circles by touching the tip of each index finger to the tip of each thumb. This subtle hand feature is called the OM mudra, and it symbolizes the merging of self with the Universe, representing serenity and divine harmony.

2. Close your eyes.

3. Focus on your breathing and take deep long inspirations through your nose and expirations through your mouth. As you are doing this, try to relax all the muscles in your body starting with your toes and methodically moving up to your head as described in the meditation in chapter three.

4. Once you are sufficiently relaxed, imagine a huge ball of bright white or yellow light above you. Feel that illuminating energy permeate warmth and tranquility throughout every cell of your body. As you breathe, inhale and absorb the bright, loving, healthy, incandescent, celestial, and vital light and exhale and expel any dark, murky, heavy, thick, or toxic energy. Picture your body and the area surrounding you warm and aglow with this light. You may even perceive that the distinctions between your body and the surrounding environment are becoming less clear as if you are becoming one with it.

5. Periodically gently rub your palms together to enhance your energy frequency.

6. Continue to focus on your breathing and the bright light for about twenty minutes. Know that this white or golden light is your connection to a higher source and that this illumination is also helping to raise your vibration as you become a conduit for the intended focus and recipient of your meditation. The healing that you request can come either during or after the meditation. The pain or trouble may be lessened or a pertinent healing message may come to you as a sudden thought, feeling, vision, or voice. Try to be open and receptive to any delivered relevant information.

7. Try not to let your mind wander. In other words, try not to think about all the chores you have to do that day or the bills you have to pay or any worries. If intrusive thoughts or concerns do enter your mind, once you have acknowledged that they are there, kindly ask them to leave. You may creatively visualize seeing them to the door and closing it behind them or viewing them attached to a large helium balloon floating up into the sky until they are out of sight or observing them inscribed on a blackboard as you erase them away. Do whatever technique works best for you to clear your mind of distractions.

8. Another approach you can choose to help train your mind to stay calm and focused utilizes a word or short phrase called a mantra (which literally means "place to rest the mind"), spoken intermittently or continuously throughout the meditation either audibly yet softly or silently and internally. The dictum usually contains some special, holy, or inspiring connotations that aid in the clearing of the

mind such as *om* (translated from Sanskrit to symbolize the first sound or vibration of creation and of being alive and considered the sound of silence that allows you to tune out thoughts and listen to the world within or nature around you). You might formulate your own personal mantra that has particular significance to you or what you hope to achieve from meditation like the following simple phrases: "right here, right now" or "be healed." Whatever mantra you choose or even if you elect not to use one at all, do what feels right to you to help you stay connected to and get the most out of your meditation experience.

9. As the meditation is coming to a close, visualize the last of the luminescence moving in the direction where the healing is intended.

10. Slowly open your eyes, stretch your body, and rub your feet on the floor as you adjust to a more grounded state of being. You may wish to say "amen" or "thank you" or a phrase of blessing or grace.

There is no fixed protocol with regard to meditation. In time and with practice you can fine-tune and develop your very own style and format that serves you best in your healing meditations.

Negative Thoughts and Worry: The Committee in Your Head

Have you ever witnessed the infectious energy of a mob? Myriad disorganized thoughts and ideas boundlessly feed into some developing cause that would never have had the gall or power to have found a pulpit of its own accord if it were not for the brutish fervor and momentum of the herd. Surrounded by a fomenting pack, people are more likely to say and do what they would otherwise have had a more difficult time initiating and justifying on their own. All you need is one or a few agitators in a crowd and it appears as if a roller coaster has left its starting gate.

A similar scenario applies to what is referred to as the *committee in your head*. You possess equivalent insurrectionists inside your mind who have a tendency to dwell on the gloomy and adverse side of issues. For instance, you have been feeling several painful stomach cramps for the past week, and all of a sudden you are grappling with the terrifying notion that you might have stomach cancer. One member of the committee points out that your late Aunt Gertrude had those same symptoms and rapidly succumbed to that disease! Another member of the committee informs you these conditions are hereditary. Isn't Aunt Gertrude your father's sister? Still another member reminds you of the article that you read in the newspaper last week citing an increased incidence of gastric carcinoma in the last decade linked to sushi. Isn't that your favorite food, and don't you eat sushi at least twice a week?

Soon all the members of the committee jump on the bandwagon until there is no opposition. The committee members seem to be plugged into the same negative energy source that fuels fear and insecurity. Soon the worst-case scenario occupies and consumes the forefront of your mind, and it is difficult to push it away. It often permeates your emotional core and physical body. It can affect sleep patterns and eating habits, not to mention how it can aggravate preexisting conditions such as depression, neurosis, migraine headaches, stomach ulcers, angina, and so on. It is much like a cancer that needs to be expunged.

Negative thoughts can give rise to that peculiar phenomenon called worry—an absorbing, fearful, chaotic, and for the most part, nonproductive state of mind. It has a habit of consuming time and energy, both of which are spent obsessing about myriad imagined dire outcomes, the majority of which never come to pass. It is a thought process just like most for which you have been hardwired, and its presence depends on how you have conditioned your mind. You can train your mental formatting through meditation and affirmations to behave and operate in a more positive and hopeful manner, or you can let your mind run wild and potentially attach to disadvantageous thought patterns and the collective consciousness.

The truth of the matter lies in the fact that there might be some constructive rationale for thinking of an unfavorable outcome, but wallowing interminably in such a state is certainly not one of them. If negativity's sole purpose is to propel you to extract yourself from its claws, allow logic and rationality to enter your thoughts, and incite you to make a worthwhile plan of action, then its intention is justified. Short of that, it does not possess redemptive qualities. It is not the preoccupation with pessimism and worry that remedies the situation, but your determination to act in the present on any valuable insight it might offer you to minimize, avoid, stop, eradicate, or handle whatever thoughts pertaining to past events or future prospects initiated it.

Your main objective should be to focus on the present. Worry is more concerned with the past and the future. The past is over, and the future is not here. If you are currently being and doing, there is no room for worry.

What did, might, will, or never happen are not here and not now, and these past or potential events can be magnified and revitalized by a mind ill at ease. Take some deep breaths and place your worrisome thoughts out of your head. Be and act in the present. Do not let those committee members in your head stir you into a tizzy.

Negativity and worry can be contagious. As with avoiding infection, it is important to fortify your system to steer clear of any unhealthy microbes and predators. Like a con, they can insidiously entice you. Like a drug, they can be an addictive and unsound mind-altering entity. Do your best to stay away from anyone and anything that thrives on, disseminates, or bolsters those attitudes.

So basically, scrutinize the reason the committee dropped by and try not to get sucked into any pernicious maelstrom. If you feel that the message or outlook is valid, heed its warnings by calmly and rationally doing whatever you can to address and prepare for the situation as best you can. If you think the warnings or prognostications are bogus, then simply ignore them and stay calm. What would be unfortunate to do is pace, pull out your hair, sweat buckets, and wait anxiously in anticipation. Do not let the committee win. Show them who the master of the mind truly is.

Ira is a sixty-eight-year-old widower. He had just had a physical examination by his primary care doctor who recommended that he schedule a routine screening colonoscopy with a specialist. In his meticulous manner, he telephoned the gastroenterologist's office the next day to book the procedure. The receptionist informed him that when she speaks with the doctor, she will get back to him shortly with a date for his procedure. Not having heard from her for a week, he decided to call again. He thought it was odd that someone did not call him back since they had always been so responsible and efficient in the past. This time the office was closed, so he left a detailed message with the answering service. After several days he still did not receive a response. Now the committee in his head was amassing numerous negative thoughts. It surmised that the doctor was avoiding him because he had consulted with his primary care physician and learned that Ira actually had some serious life-threatening condition and decided that it would simply be better to let him be than to put him through a demanding and unnecessary procedure. It also speculated that the doctors did not think that Ira was strong enough to deal with his grave condition: telling him the truth might make matters worse. He holed up in his apartment and started to plan the rest of his time as if it were merely a matter of days or weeks. He felt alone and frightened. He did not want to speak with his children and grandchildren and cause them to worry, so he isolated himself and waited for the committee's prediction.

One week later he got a call from the gastroenterologist's office with an appointment for his colonoscopy. The secretary apologized for the delay in getting back to him. The reason for the lag was that the office had been temporarily understaffed. Ira's procedure went smoothly and the findings were normal. The committee in Ira's head had decided to write him off before his time.

Ira's committee members did him a great disservice. This poor man could have succumbed to negative thinking and worry. Still his constitution proved to be mightier than his unruly mind. What a sad and futile ending it would have been if those bleak thoughts had contributed to his demise! This scenario also emphasizes that even at an advanced age, there still can be room to grow. The Universe holds an abundance of adventures and challenges to help you evolve, and it will persist in directing them your way until you have proven that you can master them successfully.

Minding the Truth

Like the archetypal image of an angel propped up on one shoulder and the devil on the other, whom are you to believe? Your mind, sometimes the rogue, might play tricks on you in order to get what it wants even to your detriment. The mind has an energy all its own, and until it is well-trained, it might not always direct you toward the truth. Truth feels as if you already know it, but all of you at one time or another have been shrewdly deceived or manipulated by a pack of lies. Even the biblical story of Adam and Eve, an integral part of many cultures, illustrates the proverbial dilemma of whom to trust—God or the serpent. Wherein lies the truth?

Often you are faced with the difficulty of having to make a decision based upon two or more conflicting choices. Your focus should be on finding the truth no matter what short-term or uncomfortable problems may result. Ultimately, it is always better to be in light than darkness. You might be tempted to select the option that offers you less of a burden or more immediate gratification, but that one might not always be where the truth lies. Look for clarity. Examine all the relevant facts and assess whether something is being concealed or some detail does not make sense. Focusing on incongruities is sometimes where the greatest revelations are revealed. Although they can be difficult to acknowledge, pay careful attention to your feelings because they can be quite effective at perceiving truth. Experience is a powerful bearer of truth. If you have had a prior similar situation, trust what you know from that. Analyze both immediate and long-term consequences as well as all pertinent motivations. Take ample time and consideration to ponder your decision scrupulously and vigilantly. Obtaining the truth not only seems right and feels light, but it also elicits a sense of certainty and soundness. And if for whatever reason, you later discover that you did not make the veracious choice, reflect on your decision-making process to see how you might improve and evolve to arrive at the truth the next time.

Rosa, a sixteen-year-old high school student, and Joey, a nineteen-year-old neighborhood boy who had dropped out of high school to work in construction, had been dating for several months. They met at a local coffee shop where she was working part-time after school as a waitress. From their first encounter, she was smitten with his rough-hewn looks and matching personality. Neither her mother nor her brother were pleased with her choice of boyfriend and expressed their opinions to her. Marco, her older brother, was aware of Joey's reputation for womanizing, and their mother Elena sized him up as a rogue not suitable for her daughter after a brief conversation when he came to their home to take Rosa out on their first proper date.

Joey was everything she had ever dreamed of in a boyfriend. At the beginning of their relationship, Joey bestowed Rosa with the proper gallantries to make her feel special; he complimented her on her beauty, bought her nice things, and took her out to restaurants, movies, and dances. She had fallen in love with him and did not understand why her family did not like him.

But after the first several months, things changed. Rosa sensed a shift in his personality. His endearments, gifts, and their dates were less frequent. He informed her that he disapproved of her family and the excessive amount of time she spent on her schoolwork and job. She took his remarks to heart. She realized how unfairly critical of Joey her mother and brother had been and that she was spending far too much time on her studies and her job at the expense of being with him. Consequently, she quit her job, eased up on her schoolwork, and became indignant toward her family.

Unfortunately and much to her mystification, none of her actions achieved her desired effect to draw Joey closer to her. As a result, she came to the conclusion that she was not good enough for him, so she attempted to woo him by dressing more provocatively and wearing more makeup. She was determined to revive their relationship. She was unaware that Joey was not being forthright and was instead insidiously distancing himself from her.

The chill in their courtship made her yearning for Joey increase. She worshipped him and could only focus on what she deemed as her flaws as possible reasons for the shift in their relationship. Her once sweet and cheerful disposition had turned sullen and moody. Her brother informed her he had seen Joey at a nightclub dancing with and kissing other girls, but she refused to believe him. She felt that Marco was just taunting her so that she would resent and forget Joey.

During her period of discontent, Rosa developed an uncomfortable, itchy, and inflamed rash on her hands. The dermatitis at first responded nicely to topical medication, but recurred when the cream was discontinued. At first, no obvious cause of her skin rash could be discovered. Both mother and daughter were extremely disappointed that I could not uncover the source of the affliction. I then explained the discipline of channeling to them and how it might offer some insight into the origin of Rosa's infirmity; they consented to try that. The message I channeled was that Rosa was placing some man on a pedestal as a symbol of great admiration, yet this man was disrespecting, deceiving, and ignoring her. Angst of her unrequited love and esteem was spawning the rash. To cure the dermatitis and prevent it from recurring, she needed to seek the truth about her relationship and fully express and eventually release her troubled feelings.

Rosa had absolutely no idea what I was talking about, but her mother certainly did. Elena explained that Rosa's boyfriend Joey was the man on the pedestal who treated her with disrespect. Rosa did not view her situation that way. The rash, her mother, her brother, and her feelings were all trying to help her find the truth.

On her walk home from school one day, Rosa took a detour through the park. She observed two lovers making out on a park bench. When she passed by close enough to see their features, she realized that the boy was Joey. She suddenly stopped, screamed at him, and ran home crying.

Rosa had difficulty seeing the truth. It is not always presented in a straightforward manner. She knew that something did not seem right in her mind about her situation, but she could not figure out what. There were definite inconsistencies in her boyfriend's actions, attitude, and words. It was crucial for her to analyze those details and draw the right conclusions. No matter what views her family members held, it was her challenge to find the truth on her own. Her feelings tried to direct her to the truth. She pined for the bliss of the earlier times she had experienced in their courtship, yet failed to heed the advice of her subsequent more doleful feelings. The dermatitis on her hands was too obscure a physical sign for her to see the connection. Circumstances such as Rosa's train the mind to learn to ascertain the truth. In this scenario, Rosa had to see it in the most direct physical presentation to believe it. Surely, she will remember this experience and better notice the signs, symptoms, feelings, and discrepancies going forward so that she will be more mindful of the truth.

The next chapter deals with the more stirring, colorful, and vibrant realm of emotions, which also play a significant role in affecting your journey of healing.

☞ 5 ☜

Healing on an Emotional Level

The Significance and Spontaneity of Emotions

Weather, like your emotions, is something over which you do not have much control. You may awaken to sun, storm, fog, warmth, cold, or a host of other environmental conditions. In the same way, sometimes certain moods overtake your sensibilities. At times you may be overcome with surprise, anger, joy, sadness, or any number of other feelings. Just as each atmospheric state is significant and essential to demonstrate and express the earth's nature, so too are your emotions vital elements necessary to convey the state of your being. If every day were warm, clear, and full of sunshine, the soil would become arid, the crops would die, the rivers and lakes would dry up, and the planet would be in a state of disaster. You need to appreciate all the meteorological conditions, for without each one of them the earth—and you—would not survive. If all your moods were gleeful, you would also not be able to properly deal with pain, misfortune, danger, iniquity, hunger, and all life's myriad of unpredictable and demanding circumstances. Just like with the many faces of climate, you must learn to understand, value, and accept each and every one of your sentiments. They are here to stay. The sooner you get comfortable with them and can be open and willing to listen to what merits they impart, the faster you can heal and become whole.

Although it is not frequently acknowledged, the emotional segment of your psyche is indeed a major player in the journey of healing. Often it is thrown together and camouflaged under the auspices of the mind. Yet the mind deals more with rational, conceptual, and intellectual concerns, whereas this emotional player is far more stirring, moving, and passionate than reason can ever dream to be. As noted in the previous chapter, often the complete package of your being is referred to with the phrase "mind, body, and spirit," which overlooks emotions. In industrialized societies where business, technology, mechanization, alacrity, and finance are valued at a high premium, emotions do not get the recognition they deserve. Feelings are not as conducive to advancing in this type of culture, so many learn to suppress and conceal that part of their essential life force in order to be acknowledged and succeed. It is still not as acceptable for men to exhibit their emotions as openly as it is for women in most societies, although that disparity is seeing some fluctuation. With regard to authorization for psychological and psychiatric treatment in the health care industry, guidelines are more equivocal and permission is more difficult to attain than they are for other fields such as those dealing with physical systems like cardiology or orthopedics. Despite all the obstacles surrounding your feelings, the pathway to becoming whole and healthy can never be reached unless you acknowledge and welcome the more passionate sides of your nature.

Your emotions are subjective and abstract perceptions unique to each of you. You cannot see or touch them, yet you are capable of knowing what you feel or perhaps what you do not want to feel. They represent another form of expression toward people, things, or situations, and they help you cope with the varied conditions of life.

Feelings are the clearest and purest form of communication. They are the language of the soul, the most direct route to the truth. To know your truth concerning something, examine what your feelings convey. They may be difficult to perceive, but when you do acknowledge them, you will discover the truth. Truth feels as if you already know it. Communication via images or words are also effectual means to know things but can be ambiguous and misleading; they may help you understand, but they can be misinterpreted because they merely stand for an impression and can never unequivocally substitute for how you feel.

Aaron is someone whom most people in our culture would consider the epitome of a successful man. By his early thirties he had already amassed a large fortune trading in commodities. He is married to a highly successful and brilliant journalist and has two fine young sons and a wonderful city apartment as well as a country home. Aaron is hardworking, sharp, decisive, impulsive, and opinionated. He has moved up the ladder quite swiftly because he has learned how to master his trade. Everything in his life is focused on going after what he desires. He is accustomed to getting what he wants, and more often than not, he is quite effective.

In the midst of all his success, Aaron has been suffering from a chronic progressive folliculitis of his scalp for approximately eight years. This is a condition where the hair follicles become inflamed and infected. With time the hair shafts shed, the follicles scar, and patches of baldness develop. One of the most unpleasant aspects of the condition for Aaron is that he suffers from bouts of intense and unmanageable itching. He has sought the aid of many highly competent and acclaimed medical experts. Several courses of conventional and appropriate therapies have been prescribed. Each time his condition would initially respond to treatment, only to recur after several months.

Why did Aaron attract his scalp disease? As with all physical ailments, the body speaks volumes of wisdom that can reveal the deeper reasons for Aaron's scalp disorder and could more effectively lead to its cure. Aaron was simply not in touch with a plethora of feelings. Most of the time he knew exactly what he was supposed to feel and went through all the correct external displays to exemplify those emotions, but he never actually deeply experienced them. The moods he was expert at sensing and projecting were the ones that strengthened his business acumen. He was a master at feeling commanding, successful, and confident, but had difficulty getting in touch with more softhearted emotions like love, happiness, sadness, and loneliness. When his father passed away, he felt a void, but no grief. When his wife temporarily left him, he was emotionally numb as he calculated ways to lure her back. Lingering and prickling deep inside were passions that percolated to and exploded on the surface of his scalp because they had been abandoned and not felt. With every scratch of his head he metaphorically tried to appease and dismiss these passions rather than acknowledge their need for integration.

If only Aaron could comprehend that by becoming acquainted with and embracing the several slighted personalities of his psyche, he would be able to begin the process of mending his emotional as well as his physical body! It is still not too late for him to heal. If his scalp condition is not enough of a catalyst to spur him to evolve, his system is sure to find another more effective way to coax him into getting in touch with his neglected emotions. Not everyone is ready to heal; they might want to do away with their afflictions, but still not be open to seeing, accepting, and working on the deeper issues responsible for attracting them. Aaron, like most, prefers the quick fixes medical science often promises and promotes. After so many failed allopathic treatments, it would seem more prudent to search elsewhere. With the right kind of knowledge, assistance, and effort, the body has amazing abilities to heal. The time has come for Aaron to look within for them. Aaron will never be able to completely heal himself until he recognizes, accepts, and welcomes the essential feelings that he has so far slighted.

Connecting with Emotions in an Exercise: A Conference Table of Emotions

It is not unusual for many people to either disconnect from, hide, curb or disproportionally cling to particular feelings, but it is even rarer for them to naturally and appropriately face and embrace them all equitably. Many individuals are daunted by the prospect of confronting and working to resolve such an issue. Another deterrent is not knowing where to begin. Seeking the aid of trained professionals is one alternative. Support groups and self-help seminars can be effective for some people. If you are open, conscientious, and aware, another route to take is to do some research and probe deeply within oneself. All choices are valid, but the right one for you depends on your specific needs, circumstances, and style. You might even choose to take advantage of more than one option.

Whether you utilize outside assistance or not, the work is still yours to do. Someone can counsel and encourage you, but the effort and onus ultimately belong to you. It is much like engaging in physical fitness. You can hire a personal trainer to teach you, demonstrate how, and push you to utilize the correct exercises, form, weights, and machines to tone and shape your body, or you may choose to take group classes or elect to do it alone by first reading, watching videos, and questioning informed sources. But in the end, it is up to you to sweat, stretch, move, exert, and work your body if you want to reach your goals. Whichever option you choose to connect with your emotions, you must be determined, dedicated, and of strong will if you aim to be successful. This type of work is not for the feeble. On a positive note, the undertaking may prove to be quite rewarding and therapeutic.

The list of emotions can be vast or condensed. Some of you utilize a multitude of emotions, while others have a more limited repertoire. You are composed of a wide array of emotive personalities, each one special and significant in its own way. To deny, hide, or excessively cling to any one of them is the equivalent to rejecting or limiting a part of yourself. The key issue is welcoming and familiarizing yourselves with an adequate complement of them in order to navigate competently through all of life's potential circumstances. The following list outlines eight basic emotions, each of which can be further subdivided into numerous related secondary ones (a sample of which are indicated in parentheses after the primary feeling):

1. LOVE (compassion, passion, devotion, caring, empathy, attraction, infatuation, appreciation)

2. JOY (ecstasy, bliss, contentment, amusement, hope-fulness, optimism)

3. SURPRISE (shock, astonishment, wonder, confusion)

4. FEAR (anxiety, distress, panic, apprehension, dread)

5. SADNESS (hurt, anguish, loneliness, disappoint-ment, shame, grief, feebleness)

6. ANGER (rage, bitterness, disgust, frustration, irrita-tion, hatred)

7. TRUST (confidence, faith, self-esteem, pride, expectation, reliance)

8. EQUANIMITY (tranquility, relaxation, composure, patience)

An exercise that can be most helpful to familiarize and instill yourself with all your many moods is to invite them to join you at a conference table. Imagine yourself positioned at the head of the table as you greet and confer with several figures with the exact same physical features as yourself seated in chairs gathered around the table. Placed in front of each character is a card inscribed with the name of a particular emotion. On your right is seated LOVE and next to LOVE is JOY followed by SURPRISE, FEAR, SADNESS, ANGER, TRUST, and lastly, EQUA-NIMITY. If you are inclined, feel free to summon to this gathering any other emotive personalities by whom you feel challenged.

In each personality you scrutinize, you can see the sentiment in their eyes, facial expression, body language, grooming, and attire. Explore what these emotions might look like for you, but an example might be the following: LOVE has dreamy eyes, is glowing and grinning, and appears to be in such a heightened, sublime, and glorious state that nothing on earth could possibly jar it. JOY is beaming with a broad toothy smile and has eyes wide open with excitement and a body radiating exuberant energy. SURPRISE has brows lifted, eyes and mouth agape, and an overall tensed musculature. FEAR is alert, sweaty, breathing rapidly, and trembling with wide-open eyes, raised eyebrows, and strained muscles. SADNESS slouches their head and shoulders, has tears in their eyes with downturned lips, and appears lethargic and less attentive to attire and grooming. ANGER is loud, flushed, and tight-lipped with angling brows and a prominent artery pulsating on the temple. TRUST exudes an honest, kind, wise, and reassuring demeanor. And lastly, EQUANIMITY wears more neutral-colored attire and has a steady, gentle, and composed appearance regardless of its surroundings. These characters are not hard to recognize with their unique features. You can actually intuit their essence. They wear "their emotions on their sleeves." It is the task of accepting, appreciating, understanding, and befriending them all that can be challenging and difficult.

Next take the time to briefly and formally greet each member at your table. You are the host and you would like all your guests to be comfortable. Try to keep a fresh, welcoming, and unbiased mind. After you have briefly gone around the room, announce that you plan to meet each personality individually in more depth. Starting either to the right or to the left of you, kindly request each temperament to join you at the head of the table where there is an empty chair placed close to yours and distant from the others. This is an opportunity for you to have a more intimate, complete, and discerning encounter with each one of them. Think of each character as a child who wants to be cherished and acknowledged. Put yourself in their shoes and try to feel what it is like to be them. Sense their essence. Ask the appropriate questions to really get into their heads. What motivates them? What causes them to nod off? What are their likes, their dislikes? Why do they behave and feel the way they do? Which other personalities do they befriend? Under what circumstances are they most likely to be of service to you or hinder you? How can you work with them to optimize and not impede attaining your goals? What rationale can you offer as to why you should make them a valued companion? Analyze how you would feel or get along if they were never to be a part of you. Look at your needs and their needs and see if there is a way that both can be satisfied. Do not hold back with any queries or issues that might pop into your head. Now is the time to be totally blunt and sincere.

After you have exhausted all the possible inquiries that you have considered and scrutinized the responses, ask yourself if you are ready to fully embrace this part of yourself. If you are, warmly welcome that part of your personality into your inner sanctum. You have now bonded and are eternally connected comrades prepared to weather whatever relevant circumstances life puts before you. If you are not at that point yet, what else do you need to know or do to close the deal? Have new doubts or questions suddenly emerged? Do you need more time? You can always send an emotion back to the conference table and revisit that relationship at a later juncture after you have acquainted yourself with some of your other guests. Perhaps it might be worthwhile if you connect first with *compassion* and *empathy* so that they may act as intermediaries in perceiving a different side of the situation. You can always request guidance from Spirit if you have sufficiently established that link. Whatever it may be that is blocking you from befriending your moods, you should continue to work on it until you have succeeded in accepting them into your coterie. If you are unable to do so, you will never completely heal or truly be whole. Remember that this work is tough, and it is a process that can take awhile. Whether it occurs now or in the near or distant future, the amount of time it takes is inconsequential, but healing is inevitable if you persevere.

You are composed of so many diverse temperaments. You may already be on good terms with many of them. In most instances, all you need to do is to reacquaint yourselves and confirm those relationships are stable and balanced. For the others, do your best to make new friends. The benefits are sure to be awesome!

Each of your emotions resonates at its own distinct energy level. Those sentiments that are often perceived as more desirable like JOY and LOVE vibrate at a higher frequency. Those temperaments often recognized as less desirable like FEAR and SADNESS vibrate at a lower frequency. Even though most of you seek higher and lighter energy states because you tend to feel better and your lives seem to flow more smoothly, they are obviously not appropriate in all situations. In some instances like after the loss of a loved one, it would be out of place to be in a high-energy state. In that setting it is most appropriate to feel SADNESS and other pertinent temperaments by residing at a denser energy level. It is only after you have spent time immersing yourself in those emotions of a low-frequency energy level that you will be able to release them and move on to lighter energy states like EQUA-NIMITY. That is why it is important to get to know all your temperaments. You cannot move from one to the other with facility otherwise, and you risk either avoiding or clinging to certain moods and becoming blocked and confined in an emotional prison.

Consequences of Avoiding Emotions

The following scenario demonstrates the potential negative consequences of an unhealthy relationship with a feeling. Frances, a sixty-five-year-old woman, was inordinately attached to anger. She suffered from a rare, unsightly, and itchy rash called lichen planus, which had been perplexingly coming and going over the course of several years. She had sores inside her mouth and multiple small violaceous bumps over her trunk and extremities. A thorough medical workup did not reveal a cause for her condition. A common treatment, cortisone, although not usually curative for this condition, can be soothing and suppressive. She responded well to that medicine.

Since I was constantly both plagued and fascinated by the true origin of illness, I decided, with Frances's permission, to channel higher sources for the reason underlying her rare and strange affliction. I received a message that the cause of this particular outbreak related to an irate altercation she had had with a man. When I asked her if any such incident had recently occurred, she turned bright red and emphatically began to berate her ex-husband, adorning her outburst with several rude expletives. Apparently, shortly before her cutaneous eruption appeared, she had had an emotional one with the father of her daughter over the financing of their daughter's education. The outcome elicited enough wrath to spawn her rash.

Once the more profound metaphysical source of the malady was determined, the work to heal her skin was redirected toward releasing her forcibly clenched and excessively protracted anger. Unfortunately, conceding her fury at that juncture proved to be particularly difficult for Frances. For some individuals, even feelings improperly employed that essentially hold them back may provide them with a false sense of secondary gain at the same time. In Frances's case, she identified herself as a victim and was not willing to give up that position and all the moods that bolstered it. In fact, she did not feel responsible for many of the unfavorable circumstances in her life. For her it was easier to place blame on others, and in order to do that, she must express a considerable amount of requisite emotion to those she deemed culpable.

About a year later while I was consulting with a patient in an exam room, I overheard some sort of confrontation coming from the front reception area. I politely excused myself from the client I was with to find out what the commotion was about. Frances, the individual responsible for the uproar, did not agree with one of the office policies and was raising her voice to my staff. I calmly attempted to discuss the matter and defuse her temper to no avail; she darted out of the office spouting some foul language. The incident confirmed to me how much her anger was dominating her emotional repertoire. To hold on to any one feeling too rigidly and interminably and avoid releasing it and moving on can lead to a great deal of emotional as well as physical infirmity. It is important to learn to give each of your feelings the necessary amount of time and attention they need and deserve—no more and no less.

Avoiding Uncomfortable Emotions with Addiction

In a perfect setting one might be resilient, bold, and competent in dealing with life's problematic circumstances and challenges; however, the reality for many is that the distressing feelings associated with addressing them are sometimes too harsh to bear. Holding on to what soothes, numbs, or removes you from a troublesome situation is an option that some of you choose even though it may perhaps lead you further from facing the problem and reaching resolution. It is alright to take some time away from a tough matter in order to have some breathing space—some extra processing time—or even an opportunity to seek trusted guidance as long as you do not create an unhealthy diversion that might lead to additional complications. Only by eventually pressing forward in an honest, clear, dedicated, and conscious state of mind can you eventually reach a constructive outcome.

Addiction can present itself in many different scenarios. Whether it shows up as eating, gambling, sex, shopping, plastic surgery, tobacco, marijuana, alcohol, opioids, or a whole gamut of other behaviors or chemical substances, the primary problem is not the unhealthy and potentially destructive compulsion, but the underlying and often shrouded inciting matter. The focus of the problem may shift, but ultimately the primary issue as well as the addiction must be addressed.

In one respect addiction can be viewed as a camouflaged urgent plea for help. Even though the addict does need help, it can seem easier for them to choose a means to escape the situation than to seek and accept assistance to address and resolve the primary issue that elicited their insufferable emotions. Not everyone has the hopefulness, the resources, the support, or the mental fortitude to take constructive steps forward. The addict finds temporary feel-good yet destructive means to cover up the problem, but it does not go away. When aid is offered, often the addict may refuse it if he is not ready, competent, and willing to do the work of healing. Sometimes addicts may have to reach the absolute worst and lowest depth of wretchedness and desperation when they can no longer adequately neutralize the discomfort of their feelings before accepting help and beginning the recovery process. The reality is that no matter how much support is provided, ultimately the task of mending rests on the shoulders of the addict. No one else can do their reparative work or live their life for them. All the best ancillary assistance in the world can only show them the right path. At that point, the rest is up to them.

Kathy, the woman presented in chapter one who mustered a "Will to Live," had grown up as the third child in a family of five daughters of alcoholic parents. Her father was emotionally and physically abusive, and her mother was emotionally too overwhelmed to protect and buffer her children. Kathy learned to give and receive the love and attention with her sisters that she desperately craved. She never stopped hoping and praying that her parents would one day assume the warm and nurturing role she envisioned, but she began to grow resentful and enraged after constant disappointment. In her early teens she turned to drugs and alcohol to anesthetize her suffering. Not at all comfortable living with and managing her plight in a wrathful state of mind on a perpetual basis, numbing her sensibilities became her unhealthy solution and plea for help. Running from her true feelings consumed twenty-five years of her life. Only after she had reached her nadir devoid of all dignity and beyond humiliation was she ready to seek professional help and face the feelings she had kept holed up deep inside. In therapy she learned to reclaim and bare her fury and eventually feel comfortable enough to welcome those once intolerable sentiments. Recognizing their central role in her circumstances helped her move forward. She was soon able to move on to other necessary and important emotions such as acceptance, compassion, empathy, and unconditional love. Eventually she learned to view her parents in a whole new light. She had evolved enough to put herself in their shoes, feel their pain, identify with their plight, and understand their choices, while at the same time acknowledging and validating her own feelings. It was advantageous for her to deal with and perceive all that was real in her life: the good, the bad, and the ugly. Kathy certainly had every right to feel angry, but she also had every right to feel loved, content, and at peace.

Feeling Your Sexuality

One of the most integral parts of your personality lies in the fact that you are sexual beings. It is important to highlight this part of your psyche separately because it often does not get the attention it deserves and its healthy integration plays such a fundamental role in making you feel whole. It is paramount to acknowledge and embrace that essential emotional and psychological constituent of your being—to be open to expressing your sexuality and to be comfortable feeling like the sexual beings you are.

The line between sexuality as a mental and an emotional state is not a clear one. Sexuality is more than a state of mind. It is true that it relates to how you think, your orientation, but it is also connected with how you feel about yourself and toward others. Physiologically the body reveals emotions. As with your other feelings, there are a whole diverse and complex mixture of hormones that surge and stir throughout the body during those heightened as well as less intense states that cause physiological responses such as stimulating or lowering your heartbeat, causing your palms to be wet or dry, your blood pressure to rise or fall, and your respiratory rate to increase or decrease. Those passionate states do not simply refer to lovemaking but also to all the emotions that surround sexuality such as feeling attractive, desired, flirtatious, covetous, aroused, infatuated, enchanted, and just plain hot and bothered. Those sentiments have the potential to give you the confidence to wink at, banter with, or caress those you are smitten with as well as feel alluring in your bodies. Regardless of your orientation, your sexuality is but one facet—albeit a significant one—of the many members of your psyche seated at the conference table whom you need to understand, accept, embrace, and feel at ease with.

You all have sexual feelings, and it is paramount that you feel comfortable accepting and conveying that part of yourselves if you ever wish to become whole. For many it seems awkward and difficult to express that part of your psyche. It is the ultimate tabooed passion. It is often more acceptable to speak openly about your rage, fears, or anxieties not related to sexuality than it is to talk about your sexual feelings. For some there appears to be embarrassment or a stigma regarding this subject. Many of you have come by information about this part of your being surreptitiously through friends, observation, experimentation, reading, cinema, television, the internet, or offbeat sources. Many of your sexual feelings are influenced by religious as well as secular cultural mores promulgated by vacillating and disparate rules and opinions. You accrue information—some of which may seem unnatural, uncomfortable, or contradictory—from so many different sources that at times it can be stressfully overwhelming and perplexing.

On a positive note, sexuality is a topic that is now generally being discussed more openly in the home as well as being taught as part of the regular curriculum on many levels of educational systems. Beneficial printed information is available through a wide range of reputable books, periodicals, and websites. There are a host of fine counselors, doctors, and clergy who are knowledgeable, caring, nonjudgmental, and willing to be of assistance. These sources can demystify and ease the tension concerning one of the most sacred and vital parts of your being. The more educated you are about sexuality and the more opportunity you have to discuss sexuality in a safe environment, the greater the likelihood that you will become more relaxed, uninhibited, and secure about your sexual feelings.

Paul is a doctor in his early forties who has had a difficult time embracing his sexuality. Growing up in a middle-class educated family where none of the emotions, let alone sexuality, was given an open forum for expression, he learned the motto "children are to be seen and not heard" at an early age. When he was eleven years old, he was sexually abused by a group of older boys at school. Severely traumatized, he learned to repress all those hurt and bitter feelings deep inside. His next sexual exposure was at sixteen with a girl his age who afterward told him that she found the experience of kissing and caressing displeasing. Subconsciously he was sexually demoralized, frustrated, and confused and pressed forward with school and his career aspirations while for the most part abandoning his needs to develop a healthy sexual life. He did date three women during college and graduate school for short interludes, but there was always something that never felt right.

When he was in his early thirties, he met a man who played a crucial role in deconstructing all his feebly assembled concepts of what a "normal" healthy active sexual relationship should constitute. At first he was veritably blind to what was occurring. This gentleman named Vittorio was three years his senior and seemed to be many things he was not: foreign, sophisticated, dashing, self-assured, and extremely knowledgeable and open about his sexuality. They swiftly developed a friendship as well as a sexual relationship. For the first time in his life Paul enjoyed expressing his sexual nature. Unfortunately, there were two big problems. For one, Paul was not completely comfortable sharing his new life with family, friends, and the public, and Vittorio was not open about his career and his nonmonogamous lifestyle. The two were actually carrying on their relationship amid secrets. Unbeknownst to Paul until late in their relationship, Vittorio was involved in nefarious occupational practices and had lovers in several cities he frequented on business. What started out on the surface to Paul as an idyllic romance shortly turned into a mystifying and tempestuous five-and-a-half-year on-again, off-again relationship. When it finally ended, Paul was psychologically devastated.

At the time what seemed to be the most emotionally shattering and disheartening event in his life proved to be the perfect catalyst to start his journey of healing. Paul spent close to two years languishing in desolation and despair. When he had finally reached a point that he was ready to climb out of his forlorn shell, he sought help. He entered therapy. He developed a voracious appetite for self-help books. He became more comfortable with expressing his feelings and his true nature. Some of his former comrades faded from his life. He eventually gravitated toward people who shared a similar mindset and with whom he felt trust, openness, and honesty. He informed his family about his sexuality. He became more health-conscious with regard to diet and exercise, and spirituality became an important focus in his life.

By embracing his sexuality—an integral part of his emotional stock—Paul also improved the mental, physical, and spiritual components of his being. There was once a time when he blamed Vittorio for annihilating his once illusory blissful state, but he eventually evolved to a point where he could bless and thank him for being the unwitting catalyst to get him to see his situation more clearly and, as a consequence, live authentically. In the past he expended so much energy avoiding and suppressing his sexual feelings that he was never able to fully enjoy the richness of life he is now able to experience.

Learning to Embrace Your Sexuality: An Exercise

The purpose of this exercise is to help you become more comfortable with your sexuality. Referring back to the section presented earlier in this chapter entitled "A Conference Table of Emotions," visualize a plaque inscribed with the word "SEXUALITY" placed in front of an identical semblance of yourself seated at a table. Imagine sitting across from, greeting, chatting with, and getting more familiar with this personality. If you are not yet totally comfortable with this part of yourself, what would it take for you to get more relaxed with this aspect of your being? What are the obstacles holding this relationship back? What can be done to overcome them? There are no restrictions to what you can ask. This is an opportunity for you to discuss what makes you feel good, bad, or any of a host of complex emotions about your sexuality. What does this persona have to offer you? What would it be like if you rejected or ignored this part of you? What is the best thing that could happen if you were to fully welcome this personality into your life? The worst thing? What can you do to judiciously maximize the best and minimize the worst scenario? Stay calm and take all the time you need to get better acquainted and have all your queries answered. You can always request help from Spirit if you have developed that connection.

When you feel that you have gathered adequate information, ask yourself if you are ready to fully accept and appropriately embrace your sexual self. If you are, you have just integrated a most valuable and vital companion into your life. If not, there is no need for concern. Take a break to review what has transpired. It might not be the right time for the two of you to merge completely. Progress might occur more gradually. You can always revisit this process later and as many times as might be necessary. There should be no pressure or deadline. Everybody heals at their own pace and in their own time. This is not a race. This is your life, and it is a wondrous journey that plays out uniquely for each of you.

Protecting Emotional Assets

Now that you either have welcomed or are in the process of at least considering accepting more of your sensitivities, it is important to keep them secure from any untoward influences. Like your family members and friends, you desire the best for them and want them to be and feel safe and protected. It is reasonable to say that you will surely not be able to protect them from all the assaults and injuries the world may subject them to. Those wounds provide experiences and influences from which you are all able to grow, but there are certainly limits to how much abuse you can withstand before you break. There is a point at which your protective armor needs to intercede. You are all endowed with these most exquisite protective coverings. They can serve you well. You must learn to keep them polished, fortified, and accessible at all times so that they can be recruited in an instant if the need arises.

As with any natural defense, you must be aware of when the appropriate moment comes to deploy your armor. There is no need to surrender your protection, suffer unnecessarily, and assume the role of martyr. That would be an endeavor in futility. For that matter, to continuously hide behind a helmet and chain mail for fear of being attacked would never allow you to grow and press on. The cocoon stages of a life cycle are meant to be limited for good reason. The seasoned, wise, and courageous soldier is one who knows and understands just exactly how, when, and why to prepare for battle. This soldier never seeks confrontation without just cause, but is well trained to handle it under appropriate circumstances. You must learn to embrace the sagacious warrior within and learn to wear armor boldly and proudly. You have worked so hard to get where you are on your journey; it would be a tragedy to relinquish your progress.

Ari is a devoted and stellar young rabbi who has served his congregation well for the past eight years. This was his first job as a head rabbi after serving as an assistant for four years at a prominent synagogue in a different part of town. He, his wife, and their three young children have come to represent an exemplary pious, righteous, and conscientious family whose deeds and traits the bulk of parishioners have come to appreciate and respect. Not only does his wife work as a historian of Jewish art, but she also volunteers her time to support and host many benefits and holiday celebrations and participates on several committees and women's groups at the synagogue. The children—ages seven, nine, and thirteen—have all assumed responsible duties partaking in religious prayer services as well as taking active roles in Jewish youth groups and events. The rabbi is a devoted pastor, and often takes on excess work to teach and counsel his congregants. He is affable and approachable and has a most difficult time saying "no." He is always ready to help someone, and he does so with a huge smile. He takes pride and joy in teaching the children in the Hebrew school. His Sabbath and High Holiday sermons receive rave reviews and often keep parishioners' minds reeling with much insight to think about in the days to follow. He is a wonderful humanitarian, leader, fundraiser, and overall inspiration to many.

Despite the rabbi's many supporters, some members of a powerfully elite board of directors at the temple did not approve of his efforts. This assembly of detractors was difficult to please. For them the rabbi did not do enough. They felt that he needed to spend more time teaching, chairing more committees, and raising more money. This displeased group had intentionally failed to deliver a written renewal contract to the rabbi for the upcoming year. Instead they had verbally informed him that he can remain in his present position without the expected cost-of-living increase in salary he was led to believe he would receive. With all that he offered of himself and provided to his congregation, he did not expect this blow.

Rabbi Ari was indeed competent and industrious. There was little time in his schedule to take on the excess responsibility of more teaching and more committee work, but he conceded. His fundraising efforts were significant. His presence had attracted many new members to the congregation. His reputation was keenly and widely noted as one of the up-and-coming outstanding figures in the city's rabbinical circles. For the most part, his congregation treasured him.

Rabbi Ari had been attacked. After doing what he had thought was a superb job, he was now questioning his abilities. He felt that all he had achieved and stood for had been undermined. No longer did he look forward to going to work every morning. It was difficult to face his parishioners with pride. He scrutinized how he could have possibly done a better job. He felt that he had given more than 100 percent of his talents, devotion, and efforts. He was humiliated and despondent and mystified by what was transpiring.

The slings and arrows of a select, albeit powerful few had an enormous effect in threatening his self-regard. Without warning they fired their weapons and directly pierced his confidence. Had he swiftly donned his armor, he would have stood up fine against any attack. Taken off guard, instead of defending his ground, he temporarily succumbed to the council's proclamation of disapproval. But this warrior's battle was not over yet. He needed time to regroup, formulate a response, and apply his sturdy armor.

In round two, he approached the governing board with determination. He chronicled his many accomplishments as well as all the changes and improvements he had enacted as chief rabbi of the temple. He spoke with dignity and sincerity. He wanted them to be fully aware of all that he had done for the synagogue. He had profited as well. He had grown into the full-fledged rabbi he was at that point partly due to how he managed his many experiences at the shul, but also because of his unique and special skills, spirit, grit, compassion, knowledge, and wisdom. He voiced how extremely grateful he was for being given this opportunity, but that it was also imperative he receive some formal recognition for his efforts. He asked for a written contract for the next year with an appropriate amount of compensation for his work. The council refused his request. He resigned, but was not defeated. He had won back his confidence and his pride. He knew that had he stayed, it would have been without self-assurance and conviction. What kind of leader or role model could he then be to his parishioners?

With the deep void of no congregation in his life, Rabbi Ari decided to write and do some teaching at a local college while at the same time searching for a position at another temple. Approximately one year later, he secured a head rabbi position at another shul in the city. He adores his new parishioners, as they do him. Even the new governing board is pleased and impressed with his abilities. He now keeps his armor close at hand knowing he will never again allow anyone to take him off guard and deprecate him undeservedly. He is back on track fulfilling his life's purpose and all the stronger, wiser, and more skilled for having persevered successfully through an unpleasant setback.

As you have already strived to heal and master the more abstract and intangible dimensions of your essence, the spiritual, the mental, and the emotional, now it is time to explore the last frontier: the most concrete, visible, and frequently probed and scrutinized aspect of your being—the physical body.

∽ 6 ∾

Healing on a Physical Level

The Concreteness and Honesty of the Physical Body

You live in a physical dimension, a tangible and down-to-earth reality. You can see, hear, touch, smell, and taste your environment. That is the classroom from which you have learned to make sense of your world. Your corporeal structure is what anchors you to this dimension and has the distinction of being the only concrete part of your being. It holds the door through which you enter and depart this life. And what a magnificent and phenomenal structure the human body is! Its temporal connection is limited, like a magnificent suit you put on that one day may be weathered and unable to keep its shape, color, and texture fresh. For the most part, whether you are willing to admit it or not, like an old broken-in pair of boots or jeans, there can be an attached appreciation, respect, and familiarity that have developed over this long-term relationship. It is an association that has indeed taught you some valuable lessons. For instance, as a child you learn that when you place your hands near a hot stove, you can feel searing pain; as an adult, most of you either know or learn that if you ingest alcohol or inhale tobacco fumes, you may leave your body susceptible to all sorts of unhealthy consequences, physical and otherwise. How fortunate you are to have a body that strives to show you, enlighten you, and steer you in a sound direction to keep you safe and well!

The physical body is an incredible messenger conveying volumes of wise and trustworthy dispatches. You only need to learn how to decipher its code and heed its messages to truly appreciate it. It will never lead you astray. When a part of you is out of sorts or unwell and you notice some physical aberrations, the body is calling on you to somehow intercede and make some changes. There is some facet deep within your system—and perhaps not just something of a corporeal aspect—reaching out to either offer guidance or ask for help. It might relate to an issue of an emotional or mental or spiritual nature. Since you are a physical being who thrives in a physical dimension and whose most potent and major warning system resides on the physical plane, you are more likely to mind and respond to messages of a physical nature compared to those with similar intent from the other three components of your being.

Some of you may have difficulty perceiving yourself beyond the boundaries of your physical body since it can seem to be the most real and vital part of your being. The following metaphysical dictum may help clarify this matter: *Your body is in you; you are not in your body.* You can move forward in the physical plane without regard to the other dimensions of your being, but that would be a foolish choice. All four travel best together as a team, supporting each other to secure stable and healthy states. If any one of them is impaired or ignored, it becomes more strenuous for you to grow and move forward on the other levels. Emotional, mental, or spiritual troubles can have a detrimental impact on physical health. When you become aware how deeper nonphysical causes for your maladies operate, you learn how to perceive and act in prudent ways that clear those blockages and revitalize and mend your material body.

The next time you feel a pang, itch, or fever, consider that underneath the external fleshy and physiological reality there exists a deeper metaphysical reason for your symptoms. This certainly does not suggest that you ignore fixing the corporeal pathology! The human body is a sacred instrument to be cherished, cared for, and preserved at all costs, but it is also imperative to look beyond the physical plane while you simultaneously repair the hull. If you disregard the more profound sources, those issues may repeatedly knock on your door either with the very same recurring maladies—albeit possibly more severe in nature—or in some other tangible way to elicit your attention. Consider the scenario of a dam where the water pressure is too great to be held in check by its physical structure. A leak which develops in the wall of the dam is repaired by a team of engineers and technicians. However, as soon as the leak is repaired, another one arises. What was mended was only a symptom of a much greater problem. Yes, the individual leaks warrant fixing, but the more deep-rooted source of the trouble that needs to be addressed is the escalating hydraulic pressure behind the dam. Once the origin of the problem is found and repaired, the other smaller complications will also dissipate.

George is an ex-CEO of an international watch company. His parents escaped communist Russia because they desired political, economic, and religious freedom.

They found refuge and made a good life for themselves in Cuba where their son was born. George holds many fond boyhood memories growing up in a small village on the island. When he was in college, there was a shortage of wristwatches for the private sector because they were being manufactured almost exclusively for the military. One summer a wealthy shoe retailer he met was looking to buy a timepiece, and George offered to find him one of those scarce commodities. So this was how his business in timepieces began, and it became extremely successful.

As the political climate was changing in Cuba, like his parents had done before, he fled his formerly beloved homeland in search of freedom. He settled in the United States with a wife, two young children, and the paltry funds he managed to smuggle out of Cuba. Hustling to provide for his family, he started over by doing the work he knew best—selling watches. Hired by a Swiss watch company, he quickly landed more accounts than any other salesperson. In time he was able to tender enough accrued earned and borrowed capital to buy the American distribution rights to the company. Yet he did not stop there. He went on to purchase two watch companies. George epitomized the American success story!

George's conviction, ambition, resourcefulness, enthusiasm, and work ethic left meager room for developing the more empathic and poignant aspects of his personality. Strong-willed, he did not respond to nudges from his family to sit back, relax, and enjoy some of the more mundane pleasures in life, so his physical body intervened to send him those messages. In his sixties he developed and was treated for a blood disorder where his body produced too many red blood cells. Following that affliction, he suffered a severe adverse drug reaction that wiped out most of his bone marrow and necessitated several blood transfusions to keep him medically stable. To add insult to injury, his lungs became inflamed and filled with fluid, and he needed to be intubated so that adequate amounts of oxygen could be delivered to his tissues. Without assurance that he would survive, he lay comatose in the intensive care unit of the hospital for several days. Miraculously he pulled through but without the same physical fortitude he had had before. His mind was still strong and active, but his body was debilitated. No longer did he have the stamina and vitality to run his empire. With no other choice, he relinquished leadership of his company to his two sons yet observed operations remotely. But after a while his scrutiny of and yearning for his business could not be contained, and he took control of his sons' corporate moves from home like a puppeteer managing marionettes. Next gout tried to impede his actions and slow him down to no avail. After that, he was lifting some heavy equipment, and his back gave out. He was in such writhing pain that he could only be comfortable in one position with a significant amount of analgesics. Frustrated at being immobilized and doped up with narcotics, George became depressed and lost his appetite. Twenty-five pounds lighter and with another complication—uncomfortable sacral pressure ulcers—he was beginning to give up hope of ever recuperating.

The real issue was that his body, directed by his soul, was urging him to surrender the indefatigable lifestyle he once led and pursue a more subdued and introspective existence. He had reached a pinnacle and excelled in one part of his life. There was no doubt that he was a master of business. What he now needed to do was to move on and deal with some other neglected elements in his life that his soul was yearning for him to experience and attend to, but he was not paying attention to the directive dispatches his body was sending him. As a clear example, while healing from his ruptured disc and bedsores, he was conducting business on a laptop computer from his bed and developed a severe case of tendonitis in his wrist. Every ailment was sending him an evident and powerful message to desist living in the manner he once did. Behaviors that once worked well for him were now detrimental to his being. The current edict from his soul routed through his physical body was mandating him to slow down, relax, appreciate nature, enjoy more simple pleasures, share more gratifying time with his wife, get more familiar with his children and grandchildren, search for his essence outside of work, and get in touch and comfortable with other varied aspects of his personality.

Finally feeling helpless, frustrated, and defeated by all his physical woes and at his family's urging, he decided to seek counseling with a psychiatrist. This was a huge leap in the right direction for this headstrong, powerful, ambitious, independent, and successful entrepreneur. Time has yet to tell whether he will be just as triumphant in this next chapter of his life. He emerged a winner before when he was dealt other tough challenges; the latest one seems to be a particularly demanding test. The Universe has provided him with all the resources to prevail in evolving and healing. Whether he truly is willing to make the essential changes in his life is ultimately up to him.

The physical body was desperately trying to send George a powerful communiqué. When he ignored one message, he was soon presented with another and yet another. His dam is still holding despite the many leaks. George may be stubborn, but he is not dense. It is not easy to change the familiar and comfortable ways that have proven to be successful in the past even though they are no longer effectual. Like George, you are all given physical signs to make changes at particular junctures in your lives. The best way to heal and move forward is to listen and try to do the necessary work your body's dispatches are advising. At the same time do not neglect to allow the proper health care workers and/or medicines and/or surgeries to assist you.

The Enigma of Physical Pathology

It is often mystifying exactly how and why pathology manifests in the body. The following are crucial questions about disease to ponder: What elicited it to arise? Why does it choose specific organs? What are the symptoms attempting to tell you? Is there a deeper meaning behind the inflammation, the infection, the cancer, the hemorrhage, and the atrophy, or is it merely concretely and solely physiologic? Do the features of its presentation hold any specific significance or provide any clues to deciphering its messages? Is there a master code to unveil? Can it reveal the answers that hold the keys to healing? Do we really have access to this information? The mind reels as the body sends communiqués!

Your body is an exquisite, brilliantly conceived, consummately built, gloriously sacred instrument that is wiser and more profound than you might think. It exudes volumes of information as well as provides you with multitudinous forms and functions. It performs uniquely for each one of you. Even though you all belong to the same species, your physical systems are similar but not identical. For one individual, the cardiac system may have been constructed with the might of Niagara Falls, but the digestive tract may have been assembled to function as poorly as a 1959 Chevy with over 200,000 miles on the odometer. Someone else may have a sturdy respiratory system engineered like a Rolls-Royce, but defective and weak rheumatological and dermatological systems akin to the quality of a twenty-year-old dilapidated Schwinn bicycle. The infirmities usually present in the physical domain at the weakest link in your anatomy. The former individual may be more prone to suffer with gastritis, while the latter person may endure arthritis and skin rashes.

Physical pathology appearing in distinct locations of the anatomy can often be associated with corresponding specific intangible issues of a mental, emotional, or spiritual nature. If there are challenges concerning a safe and secure place to feel at home in your world, the base of the spine or the rectal area might more likely attract infirmities. Difficulties with intimacy might appear as physical pathology in the pelvic, lower vertebral, or inferior abdominal regions. Power, self-esteem, trust, and responsibility issues might arise more often as ailments in the mid spine or upper abdomen near the solar plexus. Emotional troubles pertaining to love, resentment, grief, loneliness, compassion, and forgiveness might present as afflictions in the vicinity of the upper back, shoulders, or chest. Communication and creativity issues often show up as disorders in the mouth or throat/neck region. If there are blockages around authenticity, intellect, judgment, tolerance, and honesty, areas to observe dysfunction would more likely be anatomically in the head or nervous system. If someone is having challenges with spirituality, integrity, or altruism, they might have problems with muscles, bones, or skin. Stubbornness and flexibility problems can present somatically more often in the joints. If there are problems with the feet and legs, there might be issues with stability or moving forward in your life, while pathology related to the hands and upper extremities may deal with issues involving embracing and handling tough emotions or life challenges. Of course, there are exceptions to these tenets because there are usually several variables at play, but a pattern can generally be seen associated with a locale and the nature of the underlying incorporeal issue. There are no coincidences. Things occur for a reason, and where they occur is no accident even if it literally appears to be an accident. For instance, you might fall on the ice, fracture your ankle, and be incapacitated for weeks. Lately you have been in a hurry to move forward with several poorly planned projects. Perhaps this so-called accident was your soul's way of informing you via your body to slow down and take time off to rethink, regroup, and be more flexible in how you approach your work. The pathology in the locale of the foot and joint represents issues concerning moving forward and adaptability, respectively.

There are deeper reasons for all physical maladies than just anatomical aberration. The human body, being the judicious and efficient machine that it is, is always available, instructive, and truthful in shedding light and providing wisdom. Try communicating with your body the next time you feel an ache or a spasm or experience a scrape, fall, or illness. What do you sense that your body is trying to tell you? Practice being a code breaker. Ask the afflicted anatomical area what you need to know regarding its sign or symptom. It is no coincidence that physical presentations are called signs in the medical field. They might reflect signs of a basic physical property as well as a much more profound underlying emotional, cognitive, or soul issue. The body is often attempting to get your attention about some deeper matter. It is up to you whether or not to listen, decipher the communiqué, and do the work to help heal yourself. If you have mastered communicating with Spirit (chapter three), you should have the ability to ascertain that information. Spirit can relay the message. Not only would it benefit you to inquire what part you have played in attracting affliction, but also what you can do to promote healing. You indeed have access to your very own wellspring of knowledge for any potential difficulty or breakdown. Wonders never cease in how incredibly fortunate you are to be given astounding resources to aid in restoring health.

Marie is a seventy-one-year-old unmarried woman and retired accounting executive. She is a quiet, meek, and introspective woman who minds her own business. The youngest child with six older, loud, and raucous big brothers, she made her nature apparent at an early age. She was a dainty, delicate, and sensitive young girl who feared the wild, frisky, and playful abandon of her brothers. When she was four years old, her mother, to whom she was particularly close, was stricken with cancer. Her father was occupied with his work and supporting the household and was pretty unaware of the concerns of his daughter. With her mother in and out of the hospital for the next two years before she died, Marie became even more isolated from her siblings and childhood friends. Alone and deeply sad because of her mother's absence, she also became angry and bitter at her mother for abandoning her. Too young to understand the concept of death, she retreated to her own private world and rarely spoke or expressed her feelings. Fortunately for her, a favorite aunt stayed with her during that most traumatic time and brought her up after her mother passed. The aunt adored Marie and was instrumental in prying open the shell, albeit only a sliver, that tightly encased Marie's thoughts and feelings.

Fast-forward sixty-four years to a time when Marie had developed a nodule on her parathyroid gland for which her internist had referred her to a specialist. The endocrine surgeon, in excising the nodule, had accidentally damaged one of Marie's vocal cords because the nodule was growing perilously close to it. After the surgery she was not notified of any complications even though she complained of having a terribly difficult time talking. She was merely told that her symptoms were normal after this type of surgery and her troubles would take some time to abate.

Months passed and she still found it an immense effort to vocalize, so she decided to seek a second opinion. From this doctor she discovered the truth. It was explained to her that her left vocal cord had been injured during the surgery. She would be able to talk more easily as her right vocal cord strengthened with constant practice and use, but her voice might never fully recover and be as fluid and effortless as it had been before the surgery. Speech pathology helped to fortify her voice and mitigate the weakness in her throat, but it did nothing to erase the pain and anger in her psyche concerning the deception that had been unveiled. Had her initial doctors been honest and upfront with her concerning the injury to her vocal cord, she would have been upset at first but later understood that it was an unintentional surgical complication and forgiven them. She would have been at peace with both their dedicated effort and honest admission, but there was no tranquility in her for how they behaved in covering up the facts.

When she finally confronted both her primary care doctor and surgeon, both confessed to being aware of the complication but said they did not want to upset her as they were confident that in time her voice would heal on its own. She was enraged at the two of them, but kept her feelings to herself. She left their offices feeling wronged, but without the *nerve* to express how terrible she felt about the way the events transpired. Her outrage toward them stewed in her head for close to a year until her body would have no more of it.

Marie developed an acute writhing pain and rash on the right side of her forehead, temple, cheek, and upper eyelid. She had shingles, otherwise known as a varicella zoster viral infection. The breakout had originated from a cluster of nerve tissue near one side of her skull and traveled along her nerves onto her skin. She was treated with the appropriate antiviral, anti-inflammatory, and analgesic medications as well as topical disinfectant and drying compresses and lotions. Her skin eruption healed and disappeared, but the discomfort in her nerves did not dissipate as quickly.

It was as obvious as the breakout on her face what the true cause of her shingles was. Her ability to express herself had resealed itself like a tightly shut clamshell. Her anger simply needed to be articulated. It could no longer simmer inside her. The eruption was her body's way of telling her the time was long overdue to declare her feelings before her incarcerated anger found more potent and effectual means to get its point across. Still not able to face her doctors in person, she decided to express her emotions in writing. In time, after conveying and sending her sentiments to them in a letter, her nerve pain remitted.

The way Marie manifested disease is striking on two counts. For one, her inability to clearly express her thoughts and emotions materialized as physical pathology in one of her parathyroid glands and its adjacent vocal cord—both in her throat region—the seat of communication. The parathyroid glands regulate the body's calcium and phosphorus levels. In her case, a parathyroid tumor growing dangerously close to her left vocal cord was transmitting a clear message to her voice box to become more active and express itself more emphatically or else be reconciled to the fact that it might be permanently immobilized or "calcified" like stone. Marie's body had been influenced by the superconscious (soul) part of her being to generate concrete changes with the potential to push her forward in ways that her conscious mind was not able to. Were it not for the tumor growing intimately close to the vocal cord and the injury that occurred while removing it, she would not have been forced to put more effort into her communication skills. On a second count, the resentment that stirred inside from the breach of trust with her doctors presented both in her nervous system and on her most exposed anatomy—her face. The anger seethed in her nerves, a part of her physiology expressing how one perceives and reacts to the environment, and lit up her physiognomy in bold, bright, livid red hues. She figuratively and literally needed to *face* her culprits. What significantly powerful and edifying guidance the body transmits! Her anger and communication issues had never been truly resolved since her early childhood. Fortunately for Marie, the circumstances her body presented to her were instrumental in compelling her to heal herself on levels far deeper than those manifesting in the physical realm.

Understanding Life Span

It does not seem fair when a minor or anyone who has lived what is considered an abbreviated life span prematurely leaves the physical world. From a mortal standpoint you tend to view and analyze situations mundanely and not generally from the context of a higher purpose or divine perspective. It can be mystifying to consider the reasons why the soul enters and exits the physical world. The soul has a purpose in journeying to the non-spiritual domain, and that is to experience existence and evolve in ways that it could not possibly do in its natural realm. Just as you in the concrete world need to experience mystical enlightenment, so does the soul also need to expand its earthly and corporeal repertoire. When the soul has accomplished all that it has set out to do or for any number of reasons is unable to complete all its goals in its physical incarnation, it relinquishes the body. From the soul's perspective, life is eternal; it merely moves on. It also knows that it can and most probably will return to the physical dimension to bond again with a body, if it so wishes, to either set and achieve new goals or to complete what it had not yet finished in a prior time.

You have all been given time to experience existence in your bodies. What you choose to do and how you go about undertaking it have bearing on your duration or life span. Some of those objectives do not require the lengthy time frames that others do. Some of you have not been successful in your endeavors and will return for another go in another incarnation. Do not fret. The Universe truly wants you to succeed. It continues to offer you opportunities to come back until you do accomplish your objectives, and once you do, there will be more goals and other tasks to fulfill in different lifetimes. When you are able to observe your existence from a higher perspective, you will understand more clearly that it never ends. Using a metaphor to help you understand this point from an earthly perspective, you have a tendency to focus more on the planets and not the galaxies, for the planets represent the microcosm of your limited view, whereas the galaxies symbolize the more inconceivable infinite vantage point—without beginning and without end.

Physical health status and life span are generally determined by key factors. Each one of you begins life with a unique innate corporeal constitution that was carefully selected to best deal with your specific issues and life purpose. A relevant determinant of overall health and longevity relates to the quality of your initial physical composition. There is a rough linear correlation between duration of life and the fortitude of your constitution; however, the way you conduct your life also has significant bearing on longevity. Consider the parable about the straw that breaks the camel's back. If the camel is big and strong, it may take much wear and tear or many bundles of straw to break, but if the camel is small and frail, it would take less force or smaller amounts of straw for it to collapse. On the other hand, a tiny and frail camel that plays its cards right may well outlast a robust and massive one replete with trespasses and the ravages of a deleterious lifestyle. If you follow your true life purpose in optimal mental, emotional, physical, and spiritual ways, your constitution should stay heartier longer—giving you ample time to accomplish your life goals. Yet if you stray from your aspirations and/or neglect striving for those prime states of your essence, you wear down your resilience, health, and organ systems more quickly. With repeated mishaps and just plain wear and tear over time, your somatic structure begins to deteriorate until either a partial system failure or death ultimately ensues.

So it is evident that understanding the nature of life span is complex. Many factors play a role in influencing the physical body; however, it is how well you comprehensively conduct yourself in the spiritual, mental, emotional, and physical planes that has much more to do with your physical well-being and, hence, longevity than you might have previously considered. Essentially all four dimensions of your being must work together to achieve your finest and most enduring physical state.

On that rare and devastating occurrence when a fetus, infant, or young child passes, it may seem unconscionable to fathom why such an event would happen. Certainly their limited time on earth in physical form could not have accrued enough wrongdoings or depreciation to warrant such a brief existence on this plane. The truth is that when they signed their agreement to venture here, it was merely for a brief visit. They were essentially willingly contracted as pawns for that particular lifetime, so that their life would serve as a significant, meaningful, and yet shockingly strong message to those in their sphere of influence. So as those left behind mourn and try to heal, they must try to seek comfort in knowing that their loved one has returned to the grand spiritual realm from whence they came. They must also try to reach resolution and search for the greater meaning that the departed one's life and death was meant to instill in them as a catalyst—albeit a powerful and painful one—for their growth. When they see that light, then they will understand the reason and know that their loved one did not leave the physical realm in vain and is now at peace.

Then there are those cases when someone in the midst of what seemed to be a very productive and meaningful life is suddenly and seemingly accidentally whisked away for no imaginable rational reason. Again, you must focus on a much larger picture than the narrow one you envision on the earthly plane if you are ever going to be able to make sense of the loss. That soul might have accomplished all that he or she had been requisitioned to do at that juncture. Perhaps that departed one had been promoted and summoned to a higher dimension to carry out some other vital work. And as was already expressed, the impact of their life as well as their death is meant to serve as significant potential exemplars and catalysts for growth to those whose lives they touched. To illustrate this point, if you acknowledge such widely recognized individuals from your recent history like Anne Frank, James Dean, Marilyn Monroe, Sylvia Plath, John F. Kennedy, Dr. Martin Luther King Jr., John Lennon, and Princess Diana, it becomes more apparent how their prematurely abbreviated lives left extraordinary influences on the world. Sometimes the impact of the meaning and purpose of one's life can be more significant after one is gone.

You Are Given All That You Need to Attain Your Goals

On the material plane, your body tries to direct you in the most optimal manner to fulfill your life purpose. Believe it or not, you are responsible for choosing your very own bodies—equipment, if you will—to achieve your goals. Just as James Bond is provided with all the state-of-the-art high-tech gadgets to complete his mission, so are you. Each and every body is supplied with the most well-developed and necessary parts, exactly what is needed, no more and no less, to accomplish its goals in the most fitting way. There is good reason that everyone's equipment is not produced and does not function identically. You are all assigned to separate and distinct missions. No two journeys are ever exactly the same.

If an anatomic system seems atypical in construction or performance, it is not; it has been intended that way for a purpose. You are the ones who may see yourselves with aberrations or limitations; the Universe surely does not. Whether it is the color of your skin, your height, your weight, the functioning of your ears, eyes, arms, or legs, or any other distinction you perceive regarding your body, you need to look beyond any perceived irregularities and find the key to unlock your vast and unlimited potential. You must work with what you have. You are like puzzles, and if you tenaciously persevere, you will see that all the pieces fit together perfectly and perform exactly the way they are supposed to in order to achieve your life purpose. A clear example of this point would be one of the greatest competitive swimmers of all time, Michael Phelps, who has been bestowed with a body with some surprisingly uncommon dimensions, which nevertheless proved to be most advantageous for his calling. Compared to most swimmers, his above average height of 6'4", provided him with a better glide motion for extra forward momentum in the water. His exceptionally wide arm span (6'7") for a man of his height allowed him more power to push and pull himself, like the oars on a boat. His long upper body, disproportionate to his height, equipped him with a hydrodynamic triangular torso to help him move through the water with less drag. Also, his disproportionately shorter legs gave him more power in his kick, especially in his turns at the edge of the pool. The enormous size of his hands and feet offered him an edge over other swimmers in pushing and pulling himself through the water. On top of all his other atypical attributes, he was also double-jointed, a feature which allowed him extra flexibility and a greater range of motion than most of his competitors.

How You Influence Your State of Health

Responsibility for physical damage resides with the lessee. When you signed the contract, you received your bodies in pristine condition. Give or take depreciation due to normal wear and natural chronological aging, you should end up with a highly coveted and well-broken-in vintage model with all the annoying kinks ironed out. Instead what you usually finish the lease with is an undesirable, dilapidated, poorly functioning, and distressed representation. Many of you have bought into the paradigm that this is the way things are supposed to be. If you want to reap the most benefit from and appreciate the true potential of your bodies, you need to change that conceptualization, because what you believe creates your reality.

Morris is an eighty-nine-year-old widower of five years who came to see me for his psoriasis. Not only did he express dissatisfaction with his skin, but he also complained about lower back pain, frequency of urination, fatigue, and shortness of breath. When I inquired why he thought he was suffering from all these conditions, he simply replied, "Old age. These are things you must learn to live with when you get to this stage of life." Morris is getting just what he is expecting. He has programmed his mind to tell his body just what it was supposed to do and not surprisingly, his body listened and obeyed.

Millicent, on the other hand, is a ninety-four-year-old widow with a positive attitude about life and her body. She surely gets aches and pains like the rest of us, but she does not attribute them to age. Adept at listening to her physical being, when she gets tired, she rests, and when her muscles and joints ache while or after doing her exercise routine, she either takes a break or modifies her program. She does not complain or think, "Woe is me!" Millicent does not see herself as limited either mentally or physically; she just stays upbeat and flexible in order to press on with whatever life presents. When she approaches an obstacle, she does not fret but finds a positive way to deal with it. With the experience of her many years, she has clearly found a way to maintain a healthy mind and body.

Messages from the Physical Body

As sure as you can direct, instruct, impact, and confer with your body, your body can do the same with you. It is a two-way street. Every ache, pain, wound, or transgression from an optimal state of physical well-being is indeed an attempt on behalf of your corporeal sovereign forces to guide you in a better direction—a place of more stability and ease—and it is up to you to analyze the signs and act on them.

When you attract an affliction, try to make the effort to find out why and how it occurred, for then you will have set the stage for deeper levels of healing to take place. Not until you have moved toward that comprehension can you truly mitigate, repair, or cure what ails you at the deepest level. Without your quest to ascertain more profound insight, you are in effect a collaborator—albeit for the most part an unintentional or unaware one—in manifesting your own maladies. Something significant has usually gone awry in your life—something that you may not suspect or have ignored or mismanaged—and the message provoking you to deal with it has been transferred to a site in the physical body in the form of a symptom or disorder. Since you live in a physical dimension, that is deemed the most direct way of getting your attention. When you listen and start to work on the underlying issue, you can begin to mend the physical problem at its deepest source.

How appropriate that the veritable semantic interpretation of the word *disease* signifies the absence or negation of ease! By deciphering the deeper message of your signs and symptoms, your physical essence is telling you what you need to know and do in order to restore *ease* and dismiss *dis-ease*.

Hope is a twenty-seven-year-old fashion display merchandiser working and living in Manhattan. Born one of triplets, she developed a closer kinship with her gestational sister and brother than the other members of her nuclear family, which consisted of a successful businessman father, a stay-at-home mother, a sister six years her senior, and a brother three years her senior.

When Hope was eight years old, her father moved out of the family home to live with another woman, who would later become his wife and mother of their two children. Hope retained vivid memories of her father holding her on his lap telling her that he would no longer be coming home. The father with whom she yearned to have a closer emotional connection would now be physically distant. About one month later on the eve of her debut as the lead in a third-grade rendition of *Alice in Wonderland*, Hope suffered her first seizure, which her doctors later diagnosed as epilepsy. Hence, she had her own unique "looking glass" through which to view her world. Hope was devastated that she did not get the opportunity to perform, yet delighted that the doctor told her parents that they needed to pay more attention to her.

The seizures would come and go with irregular frequency and without any identifiable cause or provocation. Hope would usually sense when they were coming through a strange tingling feeling of pins and needles over her head and upper torso of approximately twenty seconds duration before the fit, which lasted anywhere from thirty seconds to about a minute. During the convulsion she would often stop breathing and lose control of several of her bodily functions. She awoke from the seizure in fog and confusion which lasted from a few hours to an entire day. When the cloudy mental state ended, she often felt rejuvenated with a lot of energy and enthusiasm to face the world.

It is necessary to know a little more background information about this young woman to truly understand how her physical body was preaching to her. Somewhat of an unconventional seeker of truths, Hope viewed the world differently than most. She had a strong spiritual frame of mind, believed that there was more to life than the material world, and was open to exploring alternative realities. She was endowed with innate gifts that allowed her unexplained knowledge of others and a forewarning of certain events. She sought out people with similar interests such as psychics, mystics, alternative healers, and those who expressed metaphysical ideologies. She believed in spirits, mediums, karma, past lives, astrology, and the tarot. Like a fish out of water, she wondered why her thoughts were so dissimilar from those of her family, who considered her odd. Her fellow triplets accepted her peculiarities without trying to understand them. Embarrassed by her idiosyncrasies, her father thought she was detached from reality, and he did not give her the emotional support she yearned for from him. Her mother was more concerned that she would become a social misfit, and her older siblings were too busy with their own lives and issues to pay her much heed.

This young woman made the most of her distinctive qualities and circumstances. Not only was she singled out for having epilepsy but also for holding unusual and mysterious beliefs and talents. Her personality traits were also notable; she was blessed with a sweet, sensitive, outgoing, nurturing, generous, and empathic disposition. Dealing with her own difficult health, family, and acceptance issues, she did not view herself as woeful or limited, but on the contrary, felt motivated to selflessly give her support to others with problems. In her spare time she mentored disadvantaged inner-city high school students, and two weeks every summer she volunteered to work at a camp for children with serious physical illnesses and disabilities.

There were certain events in her life that laid heavy burdens on her tender and impressionable psyche. When Hope was eighteen, her mother felt it an obligatory rite of passage to have her visit a gynecologist. A naïve virgin, Hope was petrified of the experience, especially of the fact that the doctor was male. Vulnerably exposed with her feet in the stirrups and the cold metal speculum inside her, she convulsed.

At college she met a sweet sensitive small-town boy named Joe who was not of her faith. She felt a warmth and comfort with him that was rare and special. They fell in love. Her parents strongly disapproved of the relationship. When Hope's father invited the triplets and their significant others on a family vacation in the Bahamas to celebrate their collective college graduations, Joe was excluded. Hope attended the trip without him but harbored resentment toward her father for not respecting her choices. Two days into the vacation she had a seizure.

After college Hope and Joe moved to New York City where they lived together. They both found work in the retail industry: he as a product buyer for a department store and she as a sales manager in a woman's clothing boutique. Their bubble burst when Joe was fired. The event placed a heavy strain on their relationship. As supportive and understanding as Hope tried to be to Joe, she could not hold their union together. Joe dealt with his troubles by distancing himself from Hope. She sensed that he was unfaithful. The joy, safety, warmth, and love she once cherished with this man were being progressively dismantled, and she felt impotent to salvage it. Eventually Joe moved out. It was during this period that Hope's seizures returned with more frequency. She would call him in her post-convulsion foggy state secretly hoping that he would console her, make her distress and hurt disappear, and mend their relationship to the way it once was. He would dutifully always come back to support and comfort her only to leave her again once he felt she had adequately recovered. When Hope came to terms with what she perceived as the finality of their relationship, the frequency of the seizures ceased.

There was one other significant provoking reason for Hope's fitful incidents. It was important for Hope to lead a clean and healthy life. She did not like putting anything impure or toxic into her body. Her diet consisted of lots of healthy fruits, nuts, and vegetables. She did not smoke, do drugs, and rarely drank alcohol. There was one event in her early twenties at a summer camp reunion where she succumbed to peer pressure and had a martini. Her body protested with a fit. Another time she injured her lower back after lifting something heavy and was in a great deal of pain. A friend coaxed her into taking some of her prescription narcotic medication. Hope's body retaliated with a seizure. She then decided to abandon the pills and simply rest until the discomfort subsided.

Epilepsy showed its presence to Hope whenever she perceived her sensitive and vulnerable nervous system to be threatened. A delicate and easily wounded individual, her infirmity was enlisted to direct her to strengthen her armor in order to cope more effectively with the uncomfortable stresses and burdens that accompanied her life. If she was ever going to be determined and confident to pursue her unique and often misunderstood mindset and mission, she needed to empower herself. She was especially tender and fragile when it pertained to distressing situations dealing with family, loved ones, or her values. Her father's departure, his not acknowledging her boyfriend, and Joe's distancing himself from her were all traumatic events which tormented her tender young psyche. Just as disturbing was the way in which her mother pushed her to have her first gynecological exam when she was not ready. In all those circumstances, her delicate mind could not cope, thereby causing it to temporarily dissociate from her body in the form of an epileptic paroxysm.

Hope's body, like her mind, was clean and pure. Any noxious substances that entered her body and clouded her sensitive and susceptible consciousness resulted in a convulsion. She would lose control of her physical functions during attacks and, in essence, release toxins from her body. The disorder freed her from an uncomfortable and unhealthy state and guided her mind and body to a more harmonious one, even causing her to feel more refreshed and rejuvenated after the fog of the seizure had cleared.

The disease or "lack of ease" in her body was acting as a signal to alert Hope to be more pure, comfortable, fearless, hardy, and powerful. Hope does not see her illness as a limitation but as a gift of guidance. She does not ponder whether she will ever grow out of it. She conceives of it as one of the methods—albeit a mighty potent one—in which the Universe channels through her and adjusts her vibration to better understand her soul, emotions, mind, and body. She feels it is a way that the "Spirit of God" communicates with her. She looks upon ailments as "something provided to remind and teach people the importance of taking care of themselves and to really grasp the whole mind, emotion, body, and spirit connection." She states, "God taught us how to heal our own bodies. Not everyone has epilepsy, but everyone has a body that some time or in some way and for some reason will have the opportunity to channel insight and wisdom. We all need to be more grateful and gracious about our bodies." Those are inspirational words from a wise and exceptional young woman with what some might label a significant plight.

The body generates wisdom for you to access. Some of you utilize it, some of you ignore it, and others are simply unaware. The body perseveres to send you information in the form of physical signs or symptoms to urge you to deal with your issues. Do your best to decipher, listen to, and comply with your body's communiqués. These messages, camouflaged as manifestations of disease, are always on target with the intelligence and guidance to help you become the grandest version of the greatest vision of who you are.

Panaceas

Many of you would like to or do indeed believe there exists that one magic potion, cream, cleanser, pill, diet, exercise device, procedure, or elixir that will transform your bodies into the epitome of health, beauty, and vitality. You read in periodicals, discover on television and radio, view on the internet, gather from salespeople and/ or experts in the field, and hear from friends and acquaintances all sorts of information about the benefits of products and treatments and how they can turn you into the visions of your dreams. You may place an awful lot of hope in external reality instead of giving yourselves credit for being able to transmute yourselves. By no means does this suggest that all these extraneous commodities do not help, but that maybe your reliance on them might be a bit overzealous.

As a former dermatologist I was constantly being asked about the perfect beauty regimen. I often saw the desperation in the inquirer's eyes. As much as I would truly have loved to be able to endorse a product that would fulfill all their hopes and expectations, I am aware that the real transformation and healing that must first take place is one that occurs in a nonphysical way. You all have the potential within to unleash that inner radiance, health, and vigor. Life would be quite simple and easy if all that stands between you and a life of wellness, beauty, and contentment were derived exclusively from a bottle, tube, pill, device, or procedure. Beauty counters across the country are very profitable for good reason; they rely to a certain degree on pandering quixotic hope. These regimens do not work unless you have a realistic attitude and understanding of who you are and what exactly you wish to accomplish. You must approach your goals by looking inside as well as outside.

As far as diet is concerned, the headlines, publicity, and scientific information are overwhelming even to the health care community. Experts do not uniformly agree on what you should be eating. The "hot" food items of today may be tomorrow's cold leftovers. Whether you select organic, natural, low-carbohydrate, high-protein, low-fat, vegetarian, juice, gluten-free, red meat, fish, or nondairy diets, the choices are baffling. How is a person to know what to do? One suggestion is to opt for food that resonates to you. Which items feel right to your system? Experiment if necessary. It may be the only way to know for sure what works for you. Remember that you can always consult Spirit (see chapter three) if you have mastered that connection.

How food affects your health might have a lot more to do with the quality of your thoughts than the quality of your food. A quote from Brugh Joy, M.D. (Joy's Way, 1979) offers a wise and straightforward perspective regarding this concept: "Foods alone will not offer a healthy body. I believe that if you put fine food into a body with a crummy mind, you get a crummy body; but if you put crummy food into a body with expanded awareness, you get a fine body. To a greater extent than we usually realize, our state of consciousness determines the way we transmute the levels of energy represented by foods, but the opposite statement would be definitely untrue; foods do not determine the level of consciousness." In that vein, it might be wiser for you to focus on more significant matters than to preoccupy yourself over the faddishness of the latest and purported greatest diets. More important, keep in mind the power enlightened thoughts hold to elevate your vibration can also elevate the energy of the foods you ingest.

Concerning all the decisions upon which you obsess about what to put in or on or, for that matter, how to exercise and tone your bodies, it is important to reiterate the fact that no two physical human specimens are entirely the same, and what works well for one may be less suitable or perhaps unfavorable for another. You all have diverse constitutions—different types of skin, unique gastrointestinal systems, body morphologies, desires, inclinations, and a host of distinct physical, chemical, spiritual, emotional, and intellectual qualities—that make you special. Why on earth should it be assumed that there would be only one soap or one cream or one diet or one exercise routine or one acne regimen or one arthritis pill or one panacea for the masses? For good reason you have an incredible array of choices. There is not one of you who fits neatly and comfortably in the dead center of every bell curve. Variety is indeed the spice of life. As you grow to embrace your differences and individuality, you must also learn to appreciate that your particular physical needs are *your* norm which you must honor and respect. So the next time a friend or colleague touts a certain extraordinary diet or miraculous cream, keep an open mind, scrutinize, and give proper thought before impulsively jumping on the bandwagon. It might certainly be an incredible product, but whether it is incredible for you is another matter.

Monica is a thirty-five-year-old fashion designer and aspiring singer who suffers from irritable bowel syndrome and is never satisfied with the condition of her skin. She truly believes that once she finds the perfect diet, day cream, night cream, cleanser, toner, and foundation, she will be set for life. She constantly reads, studies, and follows the latest nutritional news and scientific research claiming to fortify, heal, and cleanse her body. She perpetually orders money-back-guaranteed sets of facial products from late-night television infomercials promising to transform her skin into the silky, soft, and clear complexion endorsed by testimonials. Most of the new regimens seem to work for a limited time, but for reasons not clear to her, they eventually lose their effectiveness.

Another important piece of information to know concerning Monica is that she wholeheartedly believes that she has not been able to attain the status and success she feels she deserves in her two vocations. She is both a frustrated clothing designer and singer who struggles to one day become well-known and glorified for her talents. She finds the "system" unfair and feels indignant that so many others in her industries who have attained fame and success and to whom she compares herself are, in her opinion, undeserving and without merit. She is quick to lose her temper and highly emotional. She resents those in superior positions of authority for not being able to see her brilliance and talent as clearly as she does. She suffers from an inflated ego, which has managed to frustrate her and derail her goals instead of allowing Spirit to guide her joyfully in her endeavors.

Just as she cannot possibly shine and move forward comfortably in her two callings with her current attitude, neither can her complexion nor her colon, respectively. Due to her perceived lack of recognition, she suffers from frequent jealous and irascible displays of emotion that seem to correlate temporally with her facial breakouts. Periods of frustration with her work not pressing forward smoothly and favorably correspond to her colon's unstable motion and inflammation. Her skin and her digestive tract problems reflect an all too apparent metaphor for what prevails in her life. At this juncture in her journey Monica is not able to see the more profound causes of her physical troubles. She is not ready to examine or probe the more compelling issues that lie beneath the surface of her skin or within her gut. For some people it simply seems more reassuring and convenient to place their faith in the premise that their afflictions can be remedied by ingesting the latest promoted nutriment or by applying a newly developed cream purchased via a toll-free telephone number from a late-night television infomercial.

Medicines as Friends

You are social beings, and amicable and supportive relationships are instrumental to your well-being. No individual can completely thrive alone. You depend upon each other for assistance and survival. You must choose your mates carefully for some are better suited to you than others. Different friends serve distinct needs. With some you share a close attachment and a long duration, while with others there is a more casual or short-lived connection. Relationships can be complex: some are trusting and caring, others are volatile, and still others are surprisingly unsound. Yet all are established to fulfill some particular purpose.

As far as medicines are concerned, they are much like relationships. You form a very close bond with your remedies. They serve an important function in your lives. For the most part, you could not survive or at least subsist comfortably without them. They support you through both steady and rough times. Some of you may need to develop a lifelong friendship with a medicine like insulin, while others only require a short-term acquaintance with a drug such as an antibiotic.

Even though you try to seek vital, reliable, and supportive friends, some relationships are unhealthy and might be contaminated with elements of distrust, abuse, or excessive dependence. The way you regard yourself is often the way you treat your friends. If you are generally secure with yourself, you tend to choose healthy and balanced relationships. If you live predominantly in fear, you tend to attract either those who feed those fears or ones who help you overcome them. The same holds true regarding your association with pharmaceuticals, herbs, supplements, and vitamins. If you maintain a healthy and sincere regard for or deep trust in your medicaments, they tend to replenish you with the wellness you seek. If you possess an apprehensive or unhealthy attitude toward them, they might serve you with reason to confirm your views like causing adverse effects, dependency, or inefficacy. And like those who avoid attachments and might endure loneliness, there exist an equivalent minority who abstain from therapeutic drugs and might suffer the ravages of disease instead. Granted, medicines hold potent, sacred, and healing energies, but their purpose, duration, and dosage are quite specifically designed and selected to align with the correct energy frequency of your prime state of health. When their application is appropriate, too little, too much, or none at all is not sensible. Bless, honor, and respect your medicines with the same regard as you would extend to your friends. Act judiciously toward them, and they are likely to do the same toward you.

Not everyone you encounter in your lifetime would serve your highest good to befriend. Many individuals cross your path, but only a select number will qualify to be your true friends. If you feel that those seeking association with you have the ability to enhance your existence in some way without detriment, then by all means welcome them. If, however, you unequivocally feel someone is not right, it would serve you best to decline that relationship. The same holds true regarding remedies. Just as not everyone can be your friend, not every treatment will do you good. By all means trust your intuition if it is clearly and genuinely informing you that a particular pill, cream, or procedure would not serve your highest good.

Frieda is an eighty-seven-year-old German Jewish refugee fortunate to have received asylum in the United States in the late 1930s working as a young nanny for a family on Central Park West. The pain of the loss of her parents and sister annihilated by a brutal regime in her native land deeply affected her. During the time she was a governess, she managed to earn a degree in accounting while attending night school. After the war she sought employment in the accounting department of a large insurance company. It was there that she met the love of her life, Max, also a German Jewish refugee. Max was fifteen years her senior, and Frieda shared twenty blissful years with him until he passed away from cancer.

After Max's death, a common theme of abandonment by those she had loved and lost reverberated in her life, yet she was determined to press on independently. She had managed by herself before and was fiercely resolute to do so again. She was a forceful, self-reliant, stubborn, and fastidious woman. She directed much of her energy into her job until she retired at age sixty-five. Not one to sit around and be idle, she occupied her free time with her many sources of gratification: the symphony, the opera, the theater, the cinema, museums, fine dining, and traveling. She lived life thoroughly except for the fact that she was alone.

At eighty she developed an autoimmune bullous skin disease called pemphigoid. This is a rare, blistering, often self-limited, dermatologic disorder where the immune system attacks the area bordering the upper and the middle layers of the skin. Frieda was covered with tender large blisters all over her body. What's more, she was becoming weak and fragile and experienced several fainting episodes for which her doctors could not find a cause. Contrary to her wishes, she was placed on medication to help control the cutaneous disease. The pills were a godsend in regard to her skin, but caused her to feel moody, bloated, and out of sorts. She complained bitterly about the side effects, but every time the dosage was tapered, uncomfortable welts, blisters, and ulcers appeared on her skin. She had a love/hate relationship with her medicine—at times cursing it and calling it her "poison" and at other moments blessing it and grateful for its help. Forlorn, scared, and petulant, she no longer felt robust and independent anymore. Fortunately, right in her apartment complex she met a widow named Meghan twenty-five years her junior whom she employed to help her with shopping, cooking, visits to the doctor, walks in the park, and eventually getting around in a wheelchair.

This once pushy, demanding, and self-sufficient woman was discovering how to rely and depend on the support of others. She bonded with Meghan like the daughter or niece she never had. As she learned to accept assistance, she became more gracious, docile, and amiable.

Her eyes appeared kindhearted, her voice softened, and she smiled more. She not only stopped complaining about her medicine but actually expressed gratitude for it. Shortly after the change in her disposition, her disease went into remission. Her skin was now smooth and clear. She no longer needed the pills; their purpose in her life had been fulfilled. The disease had taught this fiercely independent and irascible woman well about trusting, respecting, appreciating, and welcoming the goodness and assistance of companions as well as medicines.

Once you have been given the information and the tools to heal yourselves on a physical, mental, emotional, and spiritual dimension, have absorbed these principles with some degree of comprehension and mastery, and have moved forward to become aware, mindful, wise, vital, and responsible individuals, it is natural for you to aspire to extend your enlightenment and healing energy to the rest of the world—the next topic to explore.

⌒ 7 ⌒

Healing on a Global Level

Healing as an Endless and Unique Journey

Healing never ends. Although you have walked on the moon and sent spaceships to Mars, there will always be more planets, stars, and galaxies to discover and explore in outer space. The mission of healing is as vast and infinite an endeavor as traveling throughout the cosmos. It is an endless journey of discovery, effort, change, growth, creation, and advancement. You will never arrive at your final destination. What makes the voyage so amazing is that once you have reached certain goals, there will always be other greater ones to aim for and accomplish. There will always be something more to heal. You are and always will be works in progress.

No two journeys of healing are ever the same. Everyone deals with the same issues—just at different times and in different ways. No one is ever on the same exact schedule or track or has identical circumstances. It is necessary to appreciate those distinctions and your own individual pacing. The ways you approach how you heal are also unique for each of you. If you consider climbing to the top of a mountain as a metaphor for determining how to reach your healing objective, some of you may choose a long and winding path up the incline, while others may backtrack

179

before moving upward, and still others may select a direct route to the pinnacle. The list of possibilities goes on and on, and there are no wrong choices. Whatever selection you make is the correct one for you at that precise time and for that special set of circumstances. Any of the solitary paths you may choose holds its own significant set of opportunities for growth to eventually lead you toward the same destination. You can learn French by taking a class in French, living in France, hiring a private French tutor, listening to language tapes, watching French movies or television, or dating a French girl or guy; any way you approach the language, you still learn. Since you are all distinct in your makeup and circumstances, the learning method that feels right to you *is* right for you at that specific time and place and context. Do not be harsh on yourself, but feel confident and be supportive and kind to yourself regarding the path you have chosen.

You Are All Connected

You are all connected as part of one whole, one intelligence, one energy, and one consciousness. Consequently, when you are kind and loving to another, you are doing good for the totality, and that includes you as well. And in that same vein, when you heal yourself, you are in effect essentially healing a part of the whole—something greater and bigger than yourself. Every time someone heals, they are elevating the vibration of the planet. As more of you heal, that combined energy gets more abundant until it has a contagious effect on the masses. As one person advances, he or she assists, facilitates, and points the way for another to move forward. Every time you improve yourself or aid another to get better, you are strengthening, benefiting, and advancing the totality.

Conversely, when you are hurtful and unsympathetic toward another, you are unkind and harmful toward yourself and, in effect, also hinder and negatively impact the totality. To understand this concept, consider the analogy of how unthinkable it would be to intentionally injure or maim a part of your own physical body and how it would adversely affect you as a complete being; on the other hand, when you act to enhance any part of your physical being, your entire system benefits. Try to look at your "adversaries" as a part of you; if you do right by them, wish them well, and help them to heal, you also heal and everyone benefits. Look your foes in the eye and try to see if there is a comparable part of yourself that exists in them. It might often be an aspect of yourself you are not comfortable with and have disowned. When you are able to heal yourself by having compassion, understanding, forgiveness, and acceptance for a similar unwanted and disliked element within, you just might realize that you have no enemy to face at all.

If the very best of each of you were continuously demonstrated, the planet would function more sublimely, peacefully, contently, and effectually. You would each bring out the best in one another. The Universe doled out and cleverly dispersed all its own special gifts, talents, and resources so that you could all come together as one and work collectively to create the best of all possible worlds. The potential to produce a utopia truly does exist.

Healing One Soul at a Time

The planet is figuratively becoming smaller. In these times with the burgeoning popularity and utilization of phones, radio, television, the internet, and around-the-clock local and international news broadcasts, messages and information are relayed and available straightaway. Jet transportation has made it possible to visit distant lands in hours to days. You all have the means to be connected physically and electronically as well as emotionally, mentally, and spiritually. Your popular and conventional media sources of information unfortunately expose you to and bombard you with news of turmoil, violence, murder, rape, crime, kidnappings, injury, pillage, torture, war, greed, corruption, starvation, epidemics, environmental deterioration, and other atrocities. What's more, as much as you are repulsed and distressed, you often feel equally incompetent, powerless, and ineffectual about doing anything to ameliorate or prevent these situations. The stirring is the cause of much stress and anxiety in your everyday lives. Let's face it, sitting in an outdoor café in Peoria, Illinois, discussing the problems in the Middle East is not the most effective means of helping solve the inequities in that part of the world. What can any of you do in the course of your busy and hectic lives that would truly make a significant difference in making this planet a better place to live? You can certainly choose to devote the majority of your vital energies and efforts to support a committed cause if that is where your primary aspirations and convictions lie. That might be a wonderful fit for the visions and abilities of a select group, but it also might be quite impractical for many who firmly believe in and support those objectives but have other more pressing priorities and ambitions in their lives. Yet there is indeed a way— perhaps more possible than you might have imagined— in which each and every one of you has a vital role in helping solve such meaningful global problems effectually and responsibly.

The answer resides closer to home. It begins on your doorsteps, at your dining room tables, in your living rooms, backyards, workplaces, schools, parks, playing fields, markets, houses of worship, community centers, entertainment venues, and essentially, in all your personal environments—places where you have a potentially greater impact in making changes, setting examples, and enacting beneficial results. The headlines of all the atrocities around the world should not discourage you from dealing with the troubles and injustices in your own lives, social circles, and neighborhoods. What you do and say can have a potent effect on all those you come in contact with. Each of you holds a lot of power to affect your fellow man, the animal kingdom, and your environment either directly or, just as significantly, indirectly by acting with goodness and integrity and thereby setting an example. It can be as simple and easy as smiling at a neighbor or comforting a frightened child or assisting a blind person across the street or giving helpful provisions to the poor, sick, underprivileged or offering your seat on the bus to an elderly or disabled person or donating some time or funds to your local animal humane society or recycling your refuse. If you send out goodwill to your fellow human beings, animal friends, and the natural world in the very environments you inhabit, it is sure to make a difference to and have an impact on, not only those you personally interface with but also those exposed to the ones you have encountered.

It is like an endless chain of dominos lined up and extending around the world. The effect imparted to one can have a proliferating, promulgating, and amplifying effect on others. What you do and say in Midland, Texas, can have a far-reaching effect on people and places as distant as Kabul or Baghdad or Aleppo or Tel Aviv or Chechnya. Focus on healing yourself and your own microcosms, because every individual or group that is radiating light is capable of spreading that light far beyond its bounds. Pretty soon light can overpower the darkness, and fear can be reduced and replaced with love. You have substantial roles to play in doing your part to heal the planet. No one is exempt. By raising your own vibrational energy level, you play an essential role in collectively increasing the energy frequency of the earth. It is imperative that you all help each other because when you assist one, you serve the whole, and you benefit yourself as well.

Last Comments

The undeniable truth is that at the core of all of you is a need to heal. You may not always acknowledge it, comprehend it, or be willing to face it. Some of you are so frightened that you run and hide from what you one day will brave. Make no mistake about it: not in the same way or at the same time or pace and for some, perhaps not even in this lifetime, but you will all eventually move toward the light. It is not always a smooth journey; it can at times seem daunting and tough. It all depends on how you look at it. Yet this adventure is the only one you presently have, and it promises to be a most rewarding, exciting, challenging, brilliant, fascinating, wondrous, and meaningful one if you are willing to follow some of the basic tenets outlined in this book and stay open to transformation. Try not to view it as complicated—it is not. Sound advice is usually pure and simple. Truth feels as if you already know it. Be mindful that you are what you think, and what you think, you create, and you can create anything you set your mind to. Find solace in the fact that you are not alone. Each and every one of you has been placed on this planet to support each other and to assist the whole in forging ahead.

Utilize all available resources. There are benevolent powerful forces in the Universe always available and ready to guide, support, and propel you forward. To acknowledge and heed these influences is one of the greatest revelations that will push your existence into a new and improved harmonious state of health, joy, love, equanimity, and enlightenment. You have everything you need to embark on your journey.

Remember that you all chose your talents, gifts, physical attributes, strengths, family, friends, adversaries, lovers, teachers, opportunities, goals, and challenges to help you grow and evolve on your life's journey. You have access to a vast array of knowledge, insight, wisdom, and guidance to move forward. Make the most of your efforts to mend on all your levels of being: spiritual, mental, emotional, and physical. And remember, what benefits you also serves to aid and advance the totality, for you are all connected.

Good luck and have a most blessed and wonderful journey of healing!

Acknowledgments

I began writing *Revelations on Healing* in 2003 with the excitement and passion to share my unique combined conventional medical and nontraditional healing knowledge with the world. With so many ideas, philosophies, experiences, and case histories jumbled in my mind, I had no idea how I would organize and deliver them in a way that could be read and absorbed intelligibly. Although I had never composed something of this sort before, the writing did seem to come together, but not without the amazing help of many. Not only have there been extraordinary people but also phenomenal circumstances placed in my path that guided and influenced me to be able to deliver these messages. There are several individuals who require extra special thanks and acknowledgment for being supportive, enlightening, and instrumental in helping me make *Revelations on Healing* a reality. Without them this book could not have materialized.

I do not know where to begin to convey my gratitude for Sandra Jennings's presence in my life. She is like a wondrous deity living on the earthly plane radiating infinite amounts of light, love, and wisdom. She instilled confidence in me to share my ideas and visions with the world.

I feel privileged and honored to have studied under such gifted and learned masters as Nancy Solomon, Shulamit Elson, and Peter Roth. Much of their teachings have rubbed off on me and found their way onto the pages of *Revelations on Healing*.

I am forever indebted to the invaluable services of Patty Aquirre for all her technical and computer assistance. I still keep the Post-it note she gave me with the affirmation, "YOU CAN DO IT!" adhered to my laptop computer/word processor. If I ever needed another perfect example of the positive power of affirmations, that one would surely suffice.

I extend many thanks to Inelda Perez and Agata Tuszakowski for being awesome guardians and facilitators of the sacred healing work and for perpetually striving to keep our unconventional and cherished therapeutic sanctuary sound, safe, and nurturing. Without their superb help, I would not have been able to deliver and learn from the healing work that has contributed to the foundation for *Revelations on Healing*.

This book would not have been possible without all the patients who gave me permission to render some unexpected and unconventional healing methods: To them I am truly appreciative and indebted not only for the trust they bestowed on me but also for the enlightening lessons they taught me.

I would like to extend my gratitude to my editor at Turning Stone Press, Sara Sutterfield Winn, for her diligence, efficiency, and expertise.

Jeanette Sandor, Kerianne Desiderio, and Ari Friedman deserve much thanks for their generous and painstaking efforts to proofread and edit the manuscript. Their opinions and comments helped me fine-tune my words and express my ideas more clearly and comprehensibly.

I am especially deeply grateful to my parents, Helen and Nathaniel, for giving me the space and freedom to explore and actualize many concepts which seemed unorthodox and foreign to them. My mom is responsible for influencing me to look for the good in all situations and in every person while my dad is responsible for inspiring me to become a healer like him. One of his choice catchphrases that has had an enormous impact on me during my formative years as well as being a massive source of inspiration while writing this book is, "If you have your health, you have everything!"

My heartfelt thanks go to my dear friend Kerianne, for conceiving the idea for *Revelations on Healing* in a small and understated health food café on East Eighty-Sixth Street in the spring of 2003. It was she who initiated and pushed me to share my healing concepts via this literary journey and has supplied me with nothing short of unlimited inspiration and encouragement for this challenging and rewarding endeavor. Aristotle once said, "What is a friend? A single soul dwelling in two bodies." That epitomizes what Kerianne is to me. This book is as much a part of her as it is of me.

And finally, there are almost no words that can sincerely express the love, respect, and gratitude I have for Gordon. He is the greatest, kindest, most brilliant, most understanding, and most perfect guide, teacher, healer, and friend I could have ever imagined, wished for, and chosen to assist me. I am truly blessed and thankful for all he has done for me. This book could certainly not have manifested without his expert guidance. I hope to continue our long and treasured association, and may this book be only one of a great many more joint efforts and opportunities to actualize our passion—health and healing.

Postscript

I have taken several breaks along the course of writing this book for various reasons. In some instances, the exigencies, ebbs and flows, and opportunities for healing in my own life have interrupted my writing process. Also, as I have evolved so have the messages, and I have taken the time to rewrite and upgrade them. I suspect that they will continue to grow and advance as all healing disciplines do. Another huge change for me is that after much intense deliberation, I decided to decamp from my medical practice of twenty-nine years' duration much more prematurely than I had ever imagined I would. I felt impelled to make a change. I realized it was time to move on and contribute to the field of health in a different way. Not only have I been able to devote more time to channeling, a discipline I wholeheartedly revere, but also to writing, which is a pursuit that I have come to cherish and has afforded me the means and privilege to express my words, thoughts, insights, and experiences in *Revelations on Healing* for your edification and benefit.

About the Author

Peter Wisch was born in Brooklyn, N.Y. He received a B.A. in psychology from Northwestern University, and an M.D. from the Mount Sinai School of Medicine. He trained as a medical intern at Lenox Hill Hospital and as a resident in dermatology at Emory University School of Medicine and at the Mount Sinai School of Medicine. He spent twenty-nine years practicing dermatology in his private office in NYC while also acting as a voluntary clinical professor at the Mount Sinai School of Medicine. Because of his strong interests in channeling, metaphysical principles, and alternative healing, he has devoted time pursuing those fields of study which have formed the basis for *Revelations on Healing*. He presently channels for clients in NYC.